T0198192

Melanoma

Editor

F. STEPHEN HODI

HEMATOLOGY/ONCOLOGY CLINICS OF NORTH AMERICA

www.hemonc.theclinics.com

Consulting Editors
GEORGE P. CANELLOS
EDWARD J. BENZ Jr

February 2021 • Volume 35 • Number 1

ELSEVIER

1600 John F. Kennedy Boulevard • Suite 1800 • Philadelphia, Pennsylvania, 19103-2899

http://www.theclinics.com

HEMATOLOGY/ONCOLOGY CLINICS OF NORTH AMERICA Volume 35, Number 1
February 2021 ISSN 0889-8588, ISBN 13: 978-0-323-76483-4

Editor: Stacy Eastman
Developmental Editor: Julia McKenzie

Hematology/Oncology Clinics (ISSN 0889-8588) is published bimonthly by Elsevier Inc., 360 Park Avenue South, New York, NY 10010-1710. Months of issue are February, April, June, August, October, and December. Business and Editorial Offices: 1600 John F. Kennedy Blvd., Ste. 1800, Philadelphia, PA 19103—2899. Customer Service Office: 3251 Riverport Lane, Maryland Heights, MO 63043. Periodicals postage paid at New York, NY and at additional mailing offices. Subscription prices are $456.00 per year (domestic individuals), $1150.00 per year (domestic institutions), $100.00 per year (domestic students/residents), $480.00 per year (Canadian individuals), $100.00 per year (Canadian students/residents), $1213.00 per year (Canadian institutions) $547.00 per year (international individuals), $1213.00 per year (international institutions), and $255.00 per year (international students/residents). International air speed delivery is included in all *Clinics* subscription prices. All prices are subject to change without notice. **POSTMASTER:** Send address changes to *Hematology/Oncology Clinics of North America*, Elsevier Health Sciences Division, Subscription Customer Service, 3251 Riverport Lane, Maryland Heights, MO 63043. Customer Service (orders, claims, online, change of address): Elsevier Health Sciences Division, Subscription **Customer Service, 3251 Riverport Lane, Maryland Heights, MO 63043. Tel: 1-800-654-2452 (U.S. and Canada); 314-447-8871 (outside U.S. and Canada). Fax: 314-447-8029. E-mail: journalscustomerservice-usa@elsevier.com (for print support); journalsonlinesupport-usa@elsevier.com (for online support).**

Reprints. For copies of 100 or more, of articles in this publication, please contact the Commercial Reprints Department, Elsevier Inc., 360 Park Avenue South, New York, New York 10010-1710; Tel.: 212-633-3874, Fax: 212-633-3820, E-mail: reprints@elsevier.com.

Hematology/Oncology Clinics of North America is covered in *MEDLINE/PubMed (Index Medicus), EMBASE/ Excerpta Medica, and BIOSIS.*

Contributors

CONSULTING EDITORS

GEORGE P. CANELLOS, MD
William Rosenberg Professor of Medicine, Department of Medical Oncology, Dana-Farber Cancer Institute, Boston, Massachusetts, USA

EDWARD J. BENZ Jr, MD
Professor, Pediatrics, Richard and Susan Smith Professor, Medicine, Professor, Genetics, Harvard Medical School, President and CEO Emeritus, Office of the President, Dana-Farber Cancer Institute, Boston, Massachusetts, USA

EDITOR

F. STEPHEN HODI, MD
Department of Medical Oncology, Melanoma Division, Dana-Farber Cancer Institute and Harvard Medical School, Boston, Massachusetts, USA

AUTHORS

NICOLE L. BOLICK, MD, MPH, MS
MPH Graduate, Harvard T.H. Chan School of Public Health, Boston, Massachusetts, Preliminary Medicine Resident, Department of Internal Medicine, East Carolina University/Vidant Medical Center, Greenville, North Carolina, USA

JESSICA S.W. BORGERS, MD
Department of Medical Oncology, Netherlands Cancer Institute-Antoni van Leeuwenhoek, Amsterdam, The Netherlands

ELIZABETH I. BUCHBINDER, MD
Assistant Professor, Harvard Medical School, Dana-Farber Cancer Institute, Boston, Massachusetts, USA

RICHARD CARVAJAL, MD
Associate Professor of Medicine, Director, Experimental Therapeutics and Melanoma Service, Division of Hematology/Oncology, Columbia University Irving Medical Center, New York, New York, USA

DAVID E. FISHER, MD, PhD
Professor and Chair, Department of Dermatology, Massachusetts General Hospital, Harvard Medical School, Boston, Massachusetts, USA

ALAN C. GELLER, MPH, RN
Senior Lecturer, Department of Social and Behavioral Sciences, Harvard T.H. Chan School of Public Health, Boston, Massachusetts, USA

JOHN B.A.G. HAANEN, MD, PhD
Department of Medical Oncology, Netherlands Cancer Institute-Antoni van Leeuwenhoek, Amsterdam, The Netherlands

ALEXANDRA M. HAUGH, MD, MPH
Department of Medicine, Vanderbilt University Medical Center, Nashville, Tennessee, USA

DOUGLAS B. JOHNSON, MD, MSCI
Associate Professor of Medicine, Department of Medicine, Vanderbilt University Medical Center, Vanderbilt Ingram Cancer Center, Nashville, Tennessee, USA

LILIT KARAPETYAN, MD, MS
Hematology/Oncology Fellow, Division of Hematology/Oncology, Department of Medicine, University of Pittsburgh Medical Center, Hillman Cancer Center, Pittsburgh, Pennsylvania, USA

JOHN M. KIRKWOOD, MD
Distinguished Service Professor of Medicine, University of Pittsburgh, Usher Professor of Medicine, Dermatology and Translational Science, Melanoma Center, UPMC Hillman, Pittsburgh, Pennsylvania, USA

ROHAN MANIAR, MD
Clinical Fellow, Division of Hematology/Oncology, Columbia University Irving Medical Center, New York, New York, USA

RODRIGO RAMELLA MUNHOZ, MD
Attending Physician, Oncology Center, Hospital Sírio Libanês, São Paulo, Brazil

STEPHEN M. OSTROWSKI, MD, PhD
Instructor, Department of Dermatology, Massachusetts General Hospital, Harvard Medical School, Boston, Massachusetts, USA

MICHAEL ANDREW POSTOW, MD
Melanoma Service, Memorial Sloan Kettering Cancer Center, Weill Cornell Medical College, New York, New York, USA

APRIL K.S. SALAMA, MD
Associate Professor, Department of Medicine, Duke University Medical Center, Durham, North Carolina, USA

AHMAD A. TARHINI, MD, PhD
Departments of Cutaneous Oncology and Immunology, Moffitt Cancer Center and Research Institute, Tampa, Florida, USA

Contents

The management of melanoma significantly improved within the last 25 years. Chemotherapy was the first approved systemic therapeutic approach and resulted in a median overall of survival less than 1 year, without survival improvement in phase III trials. High-dose interferon α2b and IL-2 were introduced for resectable high-risk and advanced disease, respectively, resulting in improved survival and response rates. The anti-CTLA4 and anti–programmed death 1 monoclonal antibodies along with BRAF/MEK targeted therapies are the dominant therapeutic classes of agent for melanoma. This article provides an historic overview of the evolution of melanoma management.

Melanoma skin cancer is derived from skin melanocytes and has a high risk of metastatic spread. The era of molecular genetics and next-generation sequencing has uncovered the role of oncogenic BRAFV600E mutations in many melanomas, validated the role of ultraviolet-induced DNA mutations in melanoma formation, and uncovered many of the molecular events that occur during melanoma development. Targeted therapies and immunotherapy have dramatically improved outcomes and provided an increased rate of cure for metastatic melanoma. This article reviews the formation of melanoma, the molecular events involved in melanoma growth and metastasis, and the biology underlying resistance to melanoma therapies.

Melanoma is the most common fatal type of skin cancer and is an important and growing public health problem in the United States, Australia, New Zealand, and Europe. The mortality rate in most of the world has been rising as well, albeit slower than that for incidence. Likely due to the availability of new treatments for stage 4 melanoma, mortality rates in the United States dropped 18% from 2013 to 2016. We further describe trends in melanoma incidence and mortality, review the literature on risk factors, and provide an up-to-date assessment of population-wide screening and some of the inherent concerns.

Jessica S.W. Borgers and John B.A.G. Haanen

Cancer immunotherapy plays an important role in the treatment of patients with advanced stage melanoma. Recombinant cytokines were the first tested and approved treatments; however, due to disappointing response rates and severe toxicities, their use has significantly decreased. More recently, adoptive cell transfer therapies have shown to be a promising new treatment strategy able to induce complete and durable remissions in patients with melanoma progressive on first-line treatment. This review provides an overview of the cellular therapies (tumor-infiltrating lympho-cytes, T-cell receptor T cells, chimeric antigen receptor T cells) and cyto-kine treatments (interleukin-2 [IL-2], IL-15, IL-7, IL-10, IL-21, interferon alpha, granulocyte-macrophage colony-stimulating factor) for melanoma.

Rodrigo Ramella Munhoz and Michael Andrew Postow

The treatment landscape for patients with advanced melanoma has dramatically improved over the past decade, leading to unprecedented survival. Despite the robust activity of single-agent immune-checkpoint blockade with anti–CTLA-4 or anti–PD-1 agents, and the efficacy of tar-geted therapies capable of interrupting aberrant signaling resulting from BRAF mutations, the benefit from these therapies is not universal. Advanced understanding of immune and molecular processes underlying melanoma tumorigenesis has demonstrated the promise of combined, multidrug regimens. We discuss the currently available evidence that sup-ports using combinatorial approaches in advanced melanoma treatment and provide insights into promising new combination strategies under investigation.

HEMATOLOGY/ONCOLOGY CLINICS OF NORTH AMERICA

SERIES OF RELATED INTEREST

Surgical Oncology Clinics of North America
https://www.surgonc.theclinics.com/

THE CLINICS ARE AVAILABLE ONLINE!
Access your subscription at:
www.theclinics.com

Preface

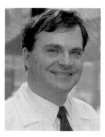

F. Stephen Hodi, MD
Editor

Over the past decade, the treatment landscape for melanoma has dramatically been altered. Improved understanding of melanoma biology, immunology, and the tumor microenvironment has transformed our abilities to provide effective therapies and translate discoveries into clinical benefits. In the past, melanoma was a disease with limited options, but now represents one of hope in becoming a chronic illness or for cure. From the targeting of driver mutations to the manipulation of immune regulation, there remains still the need for continued efforts to improve upon this elevated base of success.

In the current issue of *Hematology/Oncology Clinics of North America*, we have summoned leaders in the melanoma field to reveal its current state while providing perspective of its past and the direction of the future. Karapetyan and Kirkwood provide a historic view of the changing paradigms involving our melanoma understanding and therapeutics. Ostrowski and Fisher provide insights into the evolving melanoma biology with an emphasis on translational potential. Bolick and Geller discuss the current state of melanoma epidemiology and the changing landscape. As the novel therapeutics have demonstrated significant efficacy in the metastatic setting, Tarhini reveals the development and current use of these treatments in the adjuvant setting. Advances in our understanding and treatment of noncutaneous melanomas (ocular and mucosal) are reviewed and discussed by Carvajal and Maniar. Buchbinder highlights the critical role of immune checkpoint therapies for the treatment of melanoma. Haugh and colleagues explore the resistant mechanisms to melanoma treatments and the therapeutic roads needed to overcome such resistance. Borgers and Haanen highlight the ongoing efforts in the development of cellular therapies and cytokine treatments for melanoma. Given the number of therapeutic approaches currently available and under development, how to approach the potential for combining treatment modalities remains an important question. Munhoz and Postow discuss combinatorial approaches in the treatment of melanoma, an area that remains critical for the future of melanoma therapeutics in the hope for discovering synergistic benefits.

Hematol Oncol Clin N Am 35 (2021) ix–x
https://doi.org/10.1016/j.hoc.2020.09.006
0889-8588/21/© 2020 Published by Elsevier Inc.

We hope that this issue provides a means to advance our understanding and treat-ment of melanoma and a basis to continue efforts at improving cancer therapeutics.

F. Stephen Hodi, MD
Department of Medical Oncology
Melanoma Division
Dana-Farber Cancer Institute and
Harvard Medical School
450 Brookline Avenue
Boston, MA 02215, USA

E-mail address:
Stephen_Hodi@dfci.harvard.edu

State of Melanoma
An Historic Overview of a Field in Transition

Lilit Karapetyan, MD, MS[a], John M. Kirkwood, MD[b],*

KEYWORDS

- Melanoma • Interleukin-2 • Interferon • Immunotherapy • Targeted therapy

KEY POINTS

- The wide local excision with proper surgical margins improved morbidity and mortality of stage I/II cutaneous melanoma.
- The sentinel lymph node evaluation improved the accuracy of melanoma staging, which provides proper guidance for adjuvant therapy resulting in improved melanoma-specific survival of stage III disease.
- In patients with advanced or metastatic melanoma, systemic therapy with anti–programmed death 1 monotherapy, combination of anti–programmed death 1 and anti–cytotoxic T-lymphocyte antigen 4 monoclonal antibodies along with BRAF/MEK targeted therapy resulted in 5-year overall survival rates of 44%, 52%, and 34%, respectively.
- The fatal black tumor of the 1800s has turned into a potentially curable disease in 2020.

INTRODUCTION/HISTORY

Melanoma was first described in the literature in 1787 as a "soft and black tumor" by John Hunter. The benefit of early surgical intervention and futility of interventions later in advanced disease were well recognized in the 1800s for this "fatal black tumor," a reputation that persisted until the advent of current molecular and immunologic approaches less than 10 years ago.[1,2] The melanoma incidence rate has been increasing for generations in the United States, but age-adjusted mortality rates have fallen since 2008.[3] In 2020, 100,350 new cases of melanoma are projected, and 6850 deaths of the disease are expected in the United States.[4] These figures do not include data for melanoma in situ. The improved melanoma-specific survival and overall survival are reflections of a radical evolution in general diagnostic and management approaches over the past 25 years, that has accelerated within the last 10 years.

[a] Division of Hematology/Oncology, Department of Medicine, University of Pittsburgh Medical Center, Hillman Cancer Center, 5117 Centre Avenue, Pittsburgh, PA 15232, USA; [b] University of Pittsburgh, Melanoma Center, UPMC Hillman, Suite L1.32c Hillman Research Pavilion, 5117 Centre Avenue, Pittsburgh, PA 15232, USA
* Corresponding author.
E-mail address: KirkwoodJM@upmc.edu

Hematol Oncol Clin N Am 35 (2021) 1–27
https://doi.org/10.1016/j.hoc.2020.09.003
0889-8588/21/© 2020 Elsevier Inc. All rights reserved.

Wide local excision of the primary tumor, including proper surgical margins and the approach to regional nodes where metastasis preferentially occurs, are based on the Breslow thickness of the primary tumor, and associated with excellent survival for patients with stage I melanoma. The implementation of sentinel lymph node biopsy in patients with Breslow thickness of more than 0.76 (in the 8th edition of the American Joint Committee on Cancer [AJCC] guidelines rounded to 0.8 mm) accurately predicted risk of nodal disease approximately 10%, and potential indications for stage III disease in those with clinically occult nodal metastases, for which adjuvant immunotherapy or targeted therapy are now indicated as part of multimodality management with improved relapse-free and overall survival of patients with stage III disease.

In the 18th century, an important relationship between the immune system, infection and tumor regression were discovered after the injection of bacterial derived toxins (Coley's toxin). The role of immune surveillance was first recognized in melanoma in the late 1950s. The increased incidence of melanoma in patients with immune deficiencies, the observations of spontaneous regression of tumor and suggestions of melanoma-specific antibodies were the impetus for this hypothesis.[5–7] Intratumoral injection of BCG was reported to induce regression in up to 90% of injected sites and 17% in uninjected sites. One-fourth of patients remained disease free for up to 6 years.[8] These and the mixed bacterial vaccine of William B. Coley became a basis for the investigation of various immunotherapy approaches in the management of advanced or unresectable melanoma.

Cytokine therapy has been studied in melanoma patients across the globe since the advent of nonrecombinant and rDNA produced cytokines and interferons, resulting in responses in 10% to 20% of patients, but no rigorous evidence of an overall survival benefit. Interferon alfa-2 is the first cytokine that was identified as having benefit for the treatment of cancer. The nonrecombinant forms of interferon were initially obtained from Finnish Red Cross followed by incorporation of the industrial recombinant DNA forms in the clinical trials.[9] High doses of interferon at the maximal tolerable dosages demonstrated in phase I and II trials of the early 1980s were shown to improve disease-free and overall survival in the adjuvant setting with therapy related autoimmune findings being associated with enhanced responses. Different dosage regimens and other formulations of interferon, including pegylated interferon, were later pursued to decrease the frequency of required dosing, and to increase the exposure time. Patients with lymph node involvement and ulcerated primary melanoma were found to benefit most from both IFN alfa-2b and pegylated interferon.[10–12] In 1976, Morgan and colleagues[13] discovered a growth factor that promoted ex vivo expansion of T cells. This T-cell growth factor was termed IL-2. The role of IL-2 was investigated in advanced melanoma in multiple phase II trials over the 1990s, and resulted in durable responses in a small portion of patients.[14,15] Biochemotherapy including both IL-2 and interferon resulted in improved overall responses but evidence of improved overall survival over chemotherapy alone was elusive.[16] Toxicity related to interferon and IL-2 therapy remains the major limitation for its wide use.

Many types of vaccines including but not limited to autologous whole tumor cell vaccines such as GVAX, peptide vaccines such as MAGE-A3, gp100, ganglioside, and cellular vaccines such as Canvaxin have been widely studied in patients with melanoma. The autologous tumor-derived heat shock protein gp96 peptide complex vaccine failed to show improved survival over investigator choice therapy in patients with stage IV melanoma.[17] The ganglioside GM2 vaccine failed to show superiority over high dose interferon and observation in phase III Eastern Cooperative Oncology Group and European Organization for Research and Treatment of Cancer (EORTC) studies, respectively.[11,18] Allogeneic melanoma vaccine was tested in patients with intermediate thickness melanoma resulting in no improvement in disease free survival.[19] A polyvalent melanoma cell vaccine was pursued by several investigators to improve the overall survival of patients with stage III or IV resectable disease.[20] The follow-up studies of one of the largest phase III melanoma vaccine trials (MMAIT III/IV) unfortunately failed to show superiority of this polyvalent melanoma vaccine given with BCG, in comparison with BCG alone, in patients with resected stage III or IV melanoma. The median overall survival was 39.1 months versus 34.9 months in the BCG/placebo and BCG/CancerVax groups, respectively.[21] Unfortunately, although many vaccines demonstrated promising results in phase I and II trials the effect did not translate to overall survival benefit in large phase III trials.[22–26]

Major advancements in tumor immunotherapy stem from 1996 when the administration of immune checkpoint blockade with cytotoxic T-lymphocyte antigen 4 (CTLA-4) antibodies was shown to induce tumor regression in mouse models of melanoma.[27] In 2020, the anti–CTLA-4 and anti–programmed death 1 (PD1) monoclonal antibodies are 1 of the 2 dominant therapeutic classes of drugs for the management of melanoma.

Along with advances in immunotherapy, understanding the biology of melanoma and the role of the Ras-Raf-MEK-mitogen-activating protein-kinase (MAPK) pathway have further opened an era of targeted therapy investigation that has transformed the field of melanoma, both in patients with advanced unresectable and resectable regional disease. Presently, BRAF/MEK inhibitor combinations represent a second major class of agents for the management of melanoma. This review focuses on the historical evolution of cutaneous melanoma management, highlighting the significant advances made over the last 10 years.

EVOLUTION OF SURGICAL THERAPY

Surgery was the major therapeutic option for melanoma over the past century, and continues the mainstay of treatment for stage I or II and III resectable melanoma in 2020. The benefit of wide local excision was highlighted in the work of Samuel Cooper and William Norris in 1800s.[28] In the past, a 5-cm surgical margin was the standard of care resulting in significant skin defects, edema, and difficulties with primary closure.[29] In 1991, a World Health Organization study included patients with 2 mm and thinner melanoma and compared surgical margins of 1 cm versus greater than 3 cm. After 8 years of follow-up, the trial did not demonstrate any benefit of the larger surgical margin over 1 cm for local control of disease and overall survival.[30,31] Subsequent Swedish, French, and Intergroup studies of the surgical margin question did not reveal any local control or overall survival benefit comparing 2-cm versus 5-cm and 4-cm margins, respectively.[32–34] Another more recent Swedish study revealed no difference in overall survival comparing 2-cm and 4-cm margins.[35] After 8.8 years of follow-up, a UK study revealed improved melanoma-specific survival but failed to demonstrate overall survival benefit comparing 1-cm versus 3-cm margins in melanoma more than 2 mm in thickness.[36,37] Current guidelines recommend 0.5- to 1.0-cm surgical margins for melanoma in situ, a 1-cm margin for primary invasive melanomas of 1 mm Breslow thickness or less, and 2-cm margins for melanomas 1 to 2 mm in thickness and for those with a Breslow thickness of greater than 2 mm. Margins Trial-II is an ongoing phase III trial that compares 1-cm versus 2-cm surgical excision margins for AJCC Stage II Primary Cutaneous disease (NCT03860883).

Despite existing guidelines, surgical practice varies in the United States and in Europe and Australia. In particular, Moh's micrographic surgery is variably used among dermatologists as a surgical method for excision of cutaneous melanoma although it is not recommended in the National Comprehensive Cancer Network or American Society of Clinical Oncology guidelines, owing to concerns that the potentially narrower margins obtained may leave residual disease, owing to noncontiguous patterns of spread that are well-known in melanoma, with satellite and in-transit recurrence. Moh's micrographic surgery has been noted to increase to 7.9% in 2016 in the United States,[38] and retrospective cohort studies of approximately 70,000 patients with stage I invasive melanoma have been taken to suggest improved overall survival in the Moh's micrographic surgery cohort, but follow-up is limited and no randomized controlled study has ever rigorously established the modality of Moh's micrographic surgery.[39]

LYMPH NODE EVALUATION AND MANAGEMENT

In the 1800s, elective lymphadenectomy was proposed to prevent lymphatic dissemination of melanoma to improve the outcome for patients treated with wide surgical excision.[40] Immediate dissection of lymph nodes may have benefited patients who had occult lymph node metastases, but failed to show any benefit on overall survival.[41] This result raised the importance of determining lymph node positivity and evaluating lymph node status preoperatively to guide dissection. Lymph node evaluation techniques were published in the 1990s using radioactive tracer and the blue dye lymphazurin.[42] It became clear that primary tumor factors such as tumor thickness (>0.8 mm) and the presence of ulceration, increased number of mitoses, microsatellites, lymphovascular invasion (LVI) and absence of tumor-infiltrating lymphocytes predict the positivity of the sentinel lymph nodes.[43] The risk of lymph node involvement is less than 5% for patients with tumor thicknesses of less than 0.8 mm and goes up to 50% in stage T4b melanoma.[44] The Melanoma Institute Australia established a nomogram to predict positive sentinel lymph nodes, which include age, thickness, melanoma subtype, histology, mitoses, ulceration, and lymphatic invasion.[45]

Undoubtedly, the knowledge of sentinel lymph node status is prognostically important. In 1999, Gershenwald and colleagues[46] showed that sentinel lymph node status is the most significant prognostic factor for disease-specific survival after accounting for other clinicopathological factors of primary tumor. The Multicenter Selective Lymphadenectomy Trial (MSLT)-1 confirmed the prognostic value of sentinel lymph node biopsy in intermediate-thickness melanoma. The 5-year survival rates were 72% and 90% in patients with tumor-positive and -negative sentinel lymph nodes, respectively.[47] Subsequent 2 large trials addressed the possible benefit of complete lymph node dissection having the fact that procedure is associated with complications such as lymphedema, neuropathy, infection, and hematoma.[48,49] MSLTII revealed no melanoma-specific survival advantage of complete lymph node dissection over observation with serial ultrasound examinations in micrometastatic or clinically occult disease and resulted in a higher risk of lymphedema in the dissection group (24% vs 6%). The number of involved lymph nodes did not impact melanoma-specific survival there because involvement of nonsentinel lymph nodes was associated with poor survival in dissection group.[50] The German Dermatologic Cooperative Oncology Group trial (DeCOG-SLT) showed no improvement in recurrence-free, metastasis-free, or melanoma-specific survival after complete lymph node dissection.[51] In summary, sentinel lymph node biopsy is recommended for primary melanoma with a thickness of 0.8 mm and more; observation as opposed to complete lymph node dissection is preferred for clinically occult lymph node disease. Therapeutic lymph node dissection is recommended for clinically palpable lymph node.[52,53]

EVOLUTION OF MEDICAL THERAPY

Between 1974 and 2010, chemotherapy was the mainstay of systemic therapeutics for patients with advanced melanoma. Unfortunately, despite hundreds of trials, systemic chemotherapy resulted in no significant improvements in the survival of these patients. In 2009 based on the deliberations of the AJCC 7th classification committee, the 1-year survival rates according to M stage in the TNM system were 62%, 53% and 33% for stages M1a, M1b, and M1c melanomas, respectively.[54] There have been significant advancements in the management of advanced, unresectable, or metastatic melanoma survival over the past 10 years, following the introduction of BRAF/MEK targeted therapy, and immune checkpoint blockade with first-generation anti–CTLA-4 and second-generation anti–PD-1 and anti-PD ligand 1 therapy into clinical practice. Another approach that has achieved regulatory approval in advanced metastatic disease includes use of oncolytic viruses. To date, talimogene laherparepvec is the only oncolytic virus approved by the US Food and Drug Administration (FDA). Talimogene laherparepvec was shown to be superior to systemic granulocyte macrophage colony stimulating factor and resulted in a 16% durable response rate, with overall response rate of 26%. Response was seen in both injected and noninjected sites resulting in nonstatistically significant improved overall survival of 23 months.[55] As a result, the current five-year survival rate for patients with advanced disease approaches to 34%, 44%, and 52% in patients receiving combination of anti–CTLA-4 and anti-PD1, anti-PD1, and BRAF/MEK inhibitor therapies, respectively (**Fig. 1**).[56,57]

Adjuvant therapy is considered a standard of systemic medical management for many cancer types. Soon it started to be explored in patients with stage III or IV resected melanoma, resulting in positive outcomes in improving relapse-free survival. The presence of lymph node and/or in-transit, satellite, microsatellite metastases categorizes patient as having a stage III melanoma and is associated with worse melanoma specific and overall survival. The AJCC 8th guidelines has 4 subcategories of stage III disease accounting for characteristics of primary tumor such as thickness and ulceration, characteristics of lymph nodes including number of lymph node involved and the way of detection, and the presence or absence of satellites,

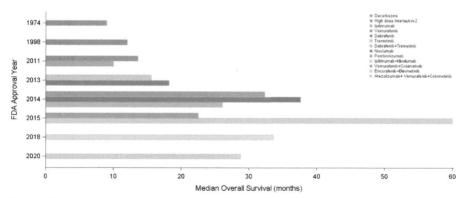

Fig. 1. Changing landscape of systemic therapy based on FDA approval timeline for advanced/metastatic melanoma. The y-axis represents year of FDA approval, the x-axis represents median overall survival (OS). The median OS improved from approximately 9 months (dacarbazine therapy) to more than 60 months. The median OS for ipilimumab and nivolumab combination therapy is more than 60 months and is not reached at the follow-up of 5 years.

microsatellites, or in-transit metastases. The new classification guides for adjuvant therapy and better stratifies patients based on recurrence risk. The survival of stage III resectable melanoma significantly improved after introduction of adjuvant therapy, and with the introduction of uniform nodal staging with sentinel node mapping and biopsy. In 2009, based on the AJCC 7th classification, the 5-year melanoma-specific survival rates for stage IIIA, IIIB, and IIIC melanoma were 78%, 59%, and 40%, respectively.[54] In 2017, based on AJCC 8th classification with uniform pursuit of sentinel lymph node biopsy, the 5-year melanoma-specific survival rates for stage IIIA, IIIB, IIIC, and IIID disease are 93%, 83%, 69%, and 32%, respectively.[44] The beneficial effect of systemic immunotherapy and targeted therapy in metastatic disease eventually moved these agents to use in the adjuvant setting as well as a standard of care therapy for stage III disease and in clinical trials for high risk stage II disease (**Fig. 2**). Among patients with a positive sentinel lymph node biopsy, the most recent change has been the abandonment of completion node dissection for patients in favor of serial ultrasound imaging after surgery on the basis of MSLTII.[50] Thus, all of the outcome data for trials before 2017, which included completion dissection for those with a positive sentinel lymph node, has changed in the past few years. We review key clinical trials for the management of advanced and stage III and IV resected disease that have led to major advancements in the field, in relation to the history of the field (**Table 1**).

1970 TO 1990: THE ERA OF CHEMOTHERAPY

Chemotherapy was the first systemic therapeutic option for the management of advanced melanoma. Dacarbazine was approved by FDA in 1974. The response to dacarbazine monotherapy varies from 5% to 28%, with a median overall survival of around 9 months and a median progression-free survival of 6 months.[58–61] Temozolomide resulted in overall response rate of 14% but did not reveal any improved overall survival or progression-free survival over dacarbazine.[58] Combination chemotherapy, including dacarbazine along with carmustine, cisplatin, and tamoxifen was not superior to dacarbazine monotherapy.[62] The altered formulation of nab-paclitaxel resulted

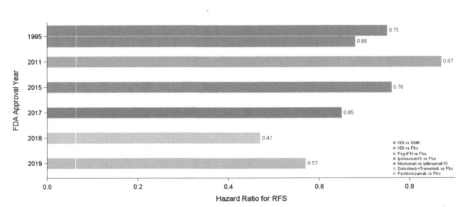

Fig. 2. Changing landscape of adjuvant therapy based on FDA approval timeline for resectable melanoma. The figure includes FDA approval year, and hazard ratio (HR) for relapse-free survival (RFS). GMK, GM2-KLH/QS-21 vaccine; HDI, high-dose interferon alfa2b; HR, hazard ratio; Ipi10, ipilimumab at 10 mg/kg dose; Pbo, placebo; PEG-IFN, pegylated interferon; RFS, relapse-free survival.

Table 1
Key findings of clinical trials in advanced/metastatic and resectable melanoma

Experimental Drug	Setting	Population (n)	Key Findings	Study/Reference
1970–1990: Chemotherapy				
DTIC	Advanced	Stage IV	ORR 15%–18% Median OS ~5–9 mo	Reviews of DTIC trials[60,61,138]
Temozolomide	Advanced	Stage IV (859)	Temozolomide did not improve PFS/ OS in comparison with DTIC Median OS ~9 mo in both group Median PFS ~2 mo in both groups	EORTRC18032[58]
1990–2010: Interferon and IL-2				
High-dose interferon α2b (HDI)	Adjuvant	Stage III (287)	HDI improved RFS and OS in comparison with placebo Median RFS 1 y→1.7 y Median OS 2.8 y→3.8 y	E1684[64]
High-dose interferon α2b Low-dose interferon α2b (LDI)	Adjuvant	Stage IIB, III (642)	HDI but not LDI improved RFS in comparison with placebo No OS difference between groups	E1690[10]
High-dose interferon α2b	Adjuvant	Stage IIB, III (880)	HDI improved RFS and OS in comparison with ganglioside vaccine GMK	E1694[11]
Pegylated interferon α2b (peginterferon)	Adjuvant	Stage III (1256)	Peginterferon improved RFS in comparison with placebo HR, 0.82 No OS difference between groups	EORTC18991[12]
High-dose IL-2	Advanced	Untreated/treated (270)	ORR 16%; CR 6% Durable responses in a portion of patients	Retrospective analysis of 8 clinical trials[14,15]

(continued on next page)

Table 1
(continued)

2010–2020: Immune checkpoint blockade and BRAF/MEK targeted therapy

Experimental Drug	Setting	Population (n)	Key Findings	Study/Reference
Ipi, 3 mg/kg;10 mg/kg	Advanced	Treated (676)	Ipi with/without gp100 is superior to gp100 HR, 0.68; 066 for median OS No difference between Ipi vs Ipi + gp100	MDX010-020[81]
	Advanced	Untreated (502)	Ipi with DTIC is superior to DTIC HR, 0.72 for 3-y OS rates	CA184-024[82]
	Advanced	Untreated (727)	Ipi 10 mg/kg is superior to 3 mg/kg but associated with higher TRAEs HR, 0.84 for median OS TRAEs 37% in Ipi10 mg/kg vs 18% in Ipi 3 mg/kg	CA184-169[84]
	Adjuvant	IIIA >1 mm IIIC 41% (Ipi) (951)	Ipi is superior to placebo HR, 0.75 for median RFS	EORTC 18071[120]
	Adjuvant	IIIB/C M1a/M1b (1670)	Ipi 3 mg/kg is superior to HDI for OS but not for RFS HR, 0.78 for OS Ipi 10 mg/kg did not result in improved OS/RFS in comparison with HDI	E1609[121]
	Advanced	Treated/untreated (834)	Pembro is superior to Ipi HR, 0.58 for 6-mo PFS HR, 0.63; 0.69 for 12-mo OS	Keynote 006[88,89]
	Adjuvant	IIIA >1 mm IIIC 38% (Pembro) (1019)	Pembro is superior to placebo Median RFS NR HR, 0.57 for 12-mo RFS	Keynote 054[123]

Drug	Setting	Population (n)	Results	Trial
Nivolumab (nivo)	Advanced	Treated (405)	Nivo resulted in higher ORR than investigator choice chemotherapy[a] (27% vs 10%) but no difference in OS	Checkmate 037[87,139]
	Advanced	Untreated (418)	Nivo is superior to DTIC HR, 0.42 for 12-mo OS	Checkmate 066[86]
	Adjuvant	IIIA Excluded IIIC 45% (Nivo) IV 18% (Nivo) (906)	Nivo is superior to Ipi Median RFS NR HR, 0.65 for 12-mo RFS	Checkmate 238[122]
Ipilimumab (ipi) plus nivolumab (nivo)	Advanced	Untreated (945)	Ipi + Nivo is superior to Ipi HR, 0.52 for median OS Increased TRAEs with Ipi/Nivo	Checkmate 067[56,91]
Vemurafenib (V)	Advanced	Untreated (675)	V is superior to DTIC HR, 0.37 for 6-mo OS HR, 0.26 for 6-mo PFS	BRIM-3[103]
	Adjuvant	IIC IIIC (cohort2) (498)	V did not improve RFS in comparison with placebo	Brim 8[124]
Dabrafenib (D)	Advanced	Untreated (733)	D is superior to DTIC HR, 0.30 for median PFS	BREAK-3[104]
Trametinib (T)	Advanced	Untreated (322)	T is superior to chemotherapy HR, 0.45 for median PFS	METRIC[105]

(continued on next page)

Table 1
(continued)

Experimental Drug	Setting	Population (n)	Key Findings	Study/Reference
Dabrafenib (D) + trametinib (T)	Advanced	Treated (247)	D + T is superior to D HR, 0.39 for median PFS Increased ORR (67% vs 51%) Decreased incidence of skin SCC (7% vs 19%)	BRF113220[140]
	Advanced	Untreated (423)	D + T is superior to D HR, 0.75 for median PFS	Combi-d[106]
	Advanced	Untreated (704)	D + T is superior to V HR, 0.69 for 1-y OS rate	Combi-v[108]
	Adjuvant	IIIA >1 mm IIIC 41% (D + T) (870)	D + T is superior to placebo HR, 0.47 for 3-y RFS	Combi-AD[125]
Vemurafenib (V) + cobimetinib (C)	Advanced	Untreated 4()95	V + C is superior to V HR, 0.51 for median PFS	coBRIM[110]
Encorafenib (E) + binimetinib (B)	Advanced	Treated/untreated (577)	E + B is superior to V HR, 0.54 for median PFS	COLUMBUS[112]
Atezolizumab + vemurafenib (V)/ cobimetinib (C)	Advanced	Untreated (514)	Atezolizumab + V/C is superior to V/C HR, 0.78 for median PFS	IMspire 150[116,117]

Abbreviations: B, binimetinib; C, cobimetinib; D, dabrafenib; DTIC, dacarbazine; E, encorafenib; HDI, high-dose interferon alfa2b; HR, hazard ratio; Ipi, ipilimumab; LDI, low-dose interferon; nivo, nivolumab; NR, not reached; ORR, overall response rate; OS, overall survival; PEG, IFN-pegylated interferon; Pembro, pembrolizumab; RFS, relapse-free survival; SCC, squamous cell cancer; T, trametinib; V, vemurafenib.

[a] Investigator choice chemotherapy: dacarbazine or carboplatin/paclitaxel.

in improved overall response rate and progression-free survival, but not overall survival in comparison with dacarbazine.[63] Dacarbazine remains the only FDA-approved chemotherapy agent for melanoma owing to a lack of evidence supporting use of other chemotherapy regimens, but it bears mention that there were never any data to indicate a survival benefit of dacarbazine therapy.

1990 TO 2010: THE ERA OF INTERFERON AND IL-2
Adjuvant Interferon Alfa-2

Following a series of studies of interferon in advanced metastatic disease that did not lead to regulatory approval, and suggested greater activity in smaller-burden disease, several trials of interferon were undertaken in the US and World Health Organization cooperative groups to determine the adjuvant role of this agent in the prevention of relapse for patients with nodal disease or deep primary melanoma at high risk of relapse. One year of high-dose interferon α2b was approved by FDA in 1995 as an adjuvant therapy for patients with stage IIB and III melanoma postoperatively. Pegylated interferon α2b was assessed in the EORTC and also approved by FDA in 2011, although no impact on survival could be shown.[12] The Eastern Cooperative Oncology Group Trial E1684 enrolled 287 patients with high-risk resected melanoma, and at median follow-up of 6.9 years revealed improvement in disease-free and overall survival in comparison with observation. Patients received IFNa2b at the dose of 20 megaunits/m² for 5 days a week for 4 weeks followed by 10 megaunit/m² subcutaneously 3 times weekly for 48 weeks. The largest benefit was noted among patients with node-positive disease.[64] In the E1690 trial, high-dose and lower dose regimens of IFN a2b were tested, and adjuvant high-dose interferon but not low-dose interferon resulted in improved relapse-free survival in comparison with observation, showing that the effect of interferon depends on the dose. Furthermore, no benefit was demonstrable in terms of overall survival in either group.[10] The superiority of adjuvant high-dose interferon therapy was reevaluated in relation to a ganglioside vaccine GMK that had been proposed by Livingston and colleagues,[65] in the E1694 trial where high-dose interferon therapy was associated with improved relapse-free (hazard ratio [HR], 1.47) and overall survival (HR, 1.52) in comparison with the GM2-KLH/QS-21 vaccine. The greatest benefit was noted in patients with node-negative disease.[11,65] The role of adjuvant high-dose interferon therapy was further explored in trials conducted in Europe in the early 2000s, with results that showed improved relapse-free survival in the Nordic trial. One Eastern Cooperative Oncology Group-led intergroup trial tested the role of the induction 1-month component of the E1684 regimen, and in E1697 the use of 1 month only of IV IFNa2b was shown not to be of benefit. A second trial that tested molecular markers of the sentinel lymph node and several other derivative aspects of interferon known as the Sunbelt trial was not performed in the cooperative groups or powered adequately to test the number of issues it addressed, and failed.[66–68] Finally, meta-analysis of various regimens using different routes, dosages, and schedules of administration demonstrated relapse-free survival and overall survival benefit with an HR of 0.87 and 0.91, respectively.[69] In overview, interferon therapy even at lower dosage and using the pegylated formulation, is associated with significant adverse effects of constitutional and flu-like toxicity, which have symptomatically limited its acceptance, along with hepatotoxicity, neurotoxicity, endocrine dysfunction, mood disorders, and thyroid dysfunction that have led to discontinuation of treatment with this drug.[70] Of interest for interferon, and is also relevant to the collateral autoimmune toxicity of later immunotherapies, the phenomena such as vitiligo and antithyroid, antinuclear, and anticardiolipin antibodies were shown to be statistically and clinically significantly associated with relapse-free survival and overall survival benefits of this therapy.[71] Owing to the adverse effect profile and its modest efficacy in comparison with current targeted and checkpoint blockade modalities, it is no longer recommended by the American Society of Clinical Oncology expert panels as a preferred choice for initial adjuvant therapy in 2020.[72]

IL-2 for the Management of Advanced, Unresectable, or Metastatic Melanoma

High-dose IL-2 was approved by the FDA in 1998 for the management of patients with metastatic melanoma on the basis of a series of phase II trials, although no phase III trial of this modality has been undertaken. The role of IL-2 in the management of cancer was extensively explored at the National Cancer Institute by Rosenberg and colleagues.[73,74] The efficacy analysis for 270 patients with metastatic melanoma enrolled in 8 clinical trials from 1985 to 1993 revealed that IL-2 resulted in an overall response rate of 16% with 6% of patients having durable complete responses.[14] The long-term follow-up of these patients confirmed durable responses in 4% of patients. The absence of disease progression was noted in all patients who had a response of more than 30 months.[15] The administration of high-dose IL-2 is associated with systemic release of inflammatory cytokines resulting in major side effects such as reversible capillary leak syndrome, fever, hypotension, cardiopulmonary, renal, and hematologic toxicities.[75–78] Despite improvement in the management of these toxicities over the years, the safety concerns along with limited efficacy in a small proportion of patients relegated high-dose IL-2 wide use to specialty units in cancer centers, and raised the unmet need for new therapeutic modalities.[79] Intratumoral IL-2 has been studied in patients with in-transit melanoma. It is well-tolerated, but responses are seen only in injected lesions.[80]

2010 TO 2020: THE ERA OF IMMUNE CHECKPOINT BLOCKADE AND TARGETED THERAPY
Anti–Cytotoxic T-Lymphocyte Antigen 4 for Management of Advanced, Unresectable, or Metastatic Melanoma

In the early 2000s anti–CTLA-4 therapy was introduced as a novel therapy for patients with metastatic melanoma. Ipilimumab was approved by the FDA in 2011 based on improved overall survival in patients with unresectable, advanced, or metastatic melanoma. In MDX010-020, the trial assessed the combination of ipilimumab at a dose of 3 mg/kg plus gp100 vaccination compared with ipilimumab and with gp100 monotherapies in second-line therapy for patients with unresectable or metastatic melanoma. Ipilimumab was associated with improved overall survival in comparison with gp100 with no difference noted between ipilimumab monotherapy and the combination. The 2-year overall survival rate was 23.5% with grade 3 and higher immune-related adverse events in up to 15% with ipilimumab therapy.[81] A second trial, MDX010-024 tested the overall survival benefit of ipilimumab at a dose of 10 mg/kg in combination with dacarbazine versus dacarbazine and showed benefit in comparison with dacarbazine monotherapy resulting in 3-year overall survival rate of 20.8%. The rate of grade 3 and higher adverse effects was 56% in the ipilimumab-containing arm.[82] The addition of granulocyte-macrophage colony-stimulating factor sargramostim to ipilimumab resulted in improved overall survival in comparison with ipilimumab monotherapy at 3 m/kg dose with median overall survival of 17.5 months versus 12.7 months in combination and monotherapy, respectively. However, progression-free survival was approximately 3 months and not different between the 2 groups.[83] This trial has been the basis of a larger phase II study that has recently graduated to stage III, in EA6141, that will be of interest in the future. Ipilimumab at a dose of

10 mg/kg was reported to be superior to the dosage of 3 mg/kg, but was associated with a higher rate of grade 3 and higher adverse effects.[84] Tremelimumab was compared with investigator choice dacarbazine or temozolomide in another large phase III trial, resulting in statistically insignificant improvements in overall survival. Despite observed overall response rates that were similar, the duration of responses was significantly longer in the tremelimumab arm (35.8 vs 13.7 months; P = .0011). Immune-related adverse effects were diarrhea, colitis, rash, and endocrine dysfunction.[85]

Anti–Programmed Death 1 for the Management of Advanced, Unresectable, or Metastatic Melanoma

Nivolumab and pembrolizumab were approved by the FDA in 2014 for the management of unresectable or metastatic melanoma. Nivolumab was associated with improved overall survival (HR, 0.42) and progression-free survival (HR, 0.43) in comparison with dacarbazine in patients with *BRAF* wild-type unresectable or metastatic melanoma as a first-line therapy. Grade 3 and higher treatment-related adverse effects were noted in only 11.7% of patients.[86] Nivolumab given as a second-line therapy for both BRAF wild-type and mutated unresectable or metastatic melanoma demonstrated durable responses (overall response rate, 31.7%), but not overall survival benefit in comparison with investigator choice chemotherapy.[87] Pembrolizumab at 2 different schedules was compared with ipilimumab, resulting in a higher overall response rate, and improved progression-free survival and overall survival.[88] This trial included both treatment-naïve patients as well as patients treated previously with *BRAF/MEK* inhibitors, chemotherapy, and immunotherapy. The 4-year overall survival rate and overall response rate were both 42% in the pooled pembrolizumab arm.[89] Patients with BRAF wild-type and with *BRAF v600 E* and *BRAF v600 K* mutation-positive melanoma, including those who were treatment naïve and who had received prior *BRAF* and/or *MEK* inhibitors, benefited from pembrolizumab therapy based on the pooled analysis of 3 major trials.[90]

Combination Therapy with Anti–Cytotoxic T-Lymphocyte Antigen 4 and Anti–Programmed Death 1 for the Management of Advanced, Unresectable, or Metastatic Melanoma

Combination therapy with nivolumab and ipilimumab was approved by the FDA in 2015 for the management of metastatic, unresectable, or advanced melanoma. CheckMate067 evaluated the role of combination therapy with ipilimumab at the dose of 3 mg/kg with nivolumab at the dose of 1 mg/kg in 1296 treatment-naïve patients with advanced disease. Nivolumab and ipilimumab resulted in an overall response rate of 58% with one-half of patients alive at 5 years. The 5-year overall survival rates were 60% and 48% in BRAF-mutated and wild-type melanoma, respectively.[56,91] The trial showed superiority of both nivolumab with ipilimumab and nivolumab monotherapy over ipilimumab monotherapy in 2 coprimary end points of progression-free survival and overall survival. Nivolumab therapy resulted in numerically lower overall response rate, progression-free survival, and overall survival in comparison with combination therapy; however, this study was not powered to detect the efficacy difference between the 2 nivolumab-containing treatment groups. The combination resulted in grade 3 and higher treatment-related adverse effects in more than one-half of the cohort, resulting in treatment discontinuation in 38% of patients owing to toxicity. The CheckMate 511 was designed to evaluate the safety of nivolumab at the dose of 3 mg/kg in combination with ipilimumab at the dose of 1 mg/kg in comparison with standard regimen. The reverse dosage of ipilimumab

(1 mg/kg) and nivolumab (3 mg/kg) combination resulted in significantly lower grade 3 and higher treatment-related adverse events at 34%. The efficacy was numerically comparable between the 2 regimens; however, the results should be interpreted cautiously because the trial was not designed to compare the efficacy outcomes.[92]

Central nervous system involvement in metastatic melanoma presents a unique therapeutic challenge with a median overall survival of 4.5 months in the early 2000s.[93] The combination of nivolumab and ipilimumab resulted the greatest efficacy reported in this cohort, demonstrating a durable response with an intracranial overall response rate of 57% and 26% with a complete response.[94,95] The combination therapy of anti-PD1 pembrolizumab with low-dose ipilimumab also showed promising results in patients with anti-PD1–refractory disease and demonstrated overall response rate of 27% and median progression-free survival of 5 months. Grade 3 and higher adverse events were reported in only 27% of patients.[96]

Targeted Therapy for Management of Advanced, Unresectable, or Metastatic Melanoma

The MAPK pathway is the major signaling pathway in the pathogenesis of melanoma.[97] In 2002, Helen Davis first described the high occurrence of somatic *BRAF* mutation in melanoma.[98] It is well-known today that 52% of cutaneous melanoma harbor *BRAF* mutation, and the most common subtypes are *V600E* followed by *V600K*.[99] The discovery of the role of *BRAF* mutation in melanoma resulted in major advancements in the management of melanoma through the intense investigation of targeted therapy directed against the MAPK pathway. Original efforts with sorafenib, a less specific RAF inhibitor, initially suggested benefit but later showed no significant impact over chemotherapy alone.[100,101] Vemurafenib was investigated in a series of trials and approved by the FDA in 2011 for the management of advanced and metastatic V600 E mutation containing melanoma. Vemurafenib resulted in overall response rate of 53% in the phase II BRIM-2 trial, and improved progression-free survival and overall survival in comparison with dacarbazine in a phase III BRIM-3 trial.[102,103] Dabrafenib was also compared with dacarbazine, resulting in improved progression-free survival and confirming the superiority of BRAF inhibitors over chemotherapy.[104] The median progression-free survival was around 5 months with single-agent BRAF inhibitors raising the need to further explore other targeted agents of MAPK pathway. The selective MEK inhibitor trametinib was compared with chemotherapy, resulting in improved progression-free survival. There were no cases of secondary skin cancers observed, but the median progression-free survival was 4.8 months.[105] *BRAF* inhibition was associated with paradoxic activation of the MAPK pathway, resulting in the development of cutaneous squamous cell carcinoma. In summary, BRAF-targeted monotherapy resulted in an increased risk of cutaneous squamous cell cancer and short progression-free survival owing to resistance to the therapy. To overcome the resistance, dabrafenib was combined with trametinib in a phase II trial and resulted in a decreased incidence of nonmelanoma cutaneous cancers and improved melanoma progression-free survival.[105] The benefit of dabrafenib plus trametinib therapy was further confirmed in 2 large phase III trials termed COMBI-v and COMBI-d, which showed both progression-free survival and overall survival benefits over BRAF monotherapy.[106–108] The pooled analysis of these 2 trials revealed 5-year progression-free survival and overall survival rates of 19% and 34%, respectively, in the dabrafenib and trametinib groups.[57] The patients with normal baseline lactate dehydrogenase level and less than 3 metastatic sites benefited the most from the dabrafenib/trametinib therapy.[109] Two other BRAF/MEK inhibitor combinations, cobimetinib with vemurafenib, and encorafenib with binimetinib, were approved by the FDA in 2015 and 2018, respectively. The cobimetinib with vemurafenib combination resulted in a median progression-free survival of 9.9 months.[110] The updated 5-year progression-free survival and overall survival rates were 14.0% and 30.8%, respectively.[111] The combination of encorafenib and binimetinib was superior to vemurafenib and encorafenib monotherapies and resulted in median progression-free survival of 14.9 months.[112,113] These 3 combinations have not been compared with each other in terms of efficacy, but they have different toxicity profiles and therapy can be changed from one to another, should specific safety concerns arise. The combination of encorafenib plus binimetinib is associated with increased γ-glutamyltransferase, creatine phosphokinase, and hypertension. Vemurafenib and cobimetinib combination is associated with pyrexia and dehydration as well as photosensitivity. Dabrafenib and trametinib therapy is associated with pyrexia, diarrhea, and arthralgia.

Targeted Therapy in Combination with Immunotherapy for the Management of Advanced, Unresectable, or Metastatic Melanoma

Targeted therapy with BRAF/MEK inhibitors is associated with increase in tumor associated antigen expression, CD8$^+$ T-cell infiltration, PD/PD ligan 1 expression and decrease in immunosuppressive cytokines such as IL-6 and IL-8.[114] The synergy of BRAF inhibition along with anti-PD1 therapy was demonstrated in a BRAFV600E syngeneic tumor graft mouse model. The combination resulted in increased numbers of tumor-infiltrating lymphocytes and enhanced responses.[115] Based on these preclinical data, the combination of *BRAF/MEK* inhibitors with anti-PD1/PD ligand 1 is being evaluated in clinical trials. Targeted therapy results in an increased response rate; however, responses are not durable. There as immunotherapy results in durable responses in some proportion of patients. The major goal of the combination of these 2 approaches is to achieve in durable responses in a large proportion of patients. The results of IMspire150 trial, which combined atezolizumab with cobimetinib and vemurafenib, were recently presented at the American Association for Cancer Research 2020 meeting and showed promising results. The triplet therapy resulted in a 54% progression-free survival rate at 12 months, an overall response rate of 66% with a median duration of response 21 months, and a median overall survival of 28.8 months. One-third of patients experienced serious therapy-related adverse effects with 12.6% of patients discontinuing trial treatment owing to toxicity. The most common adverse effects were pyrexia and arthralgia.[116,117] Based on these trial results, the FDA approved the triplet of vemurafenib, cobimetinib, and atezolizumab for *BRAFV600E/K*–mutant metastatic melanoma in July 2020 for management of advanced/metastatic disease. Despite initial promising results of combination therapy anti-PD1 inhibitor spartalizumab with dabrafenib/trametinib, the Combi-i trial did not meet the primary end point of progression-free survival.[118]

Adjuvant Immune Checkpoint Blockade Therapy

Anti–cytotoxic T-lymphocyte antigen 4
EORTC 18071 evaluated the role of 10 mg/kg adjuvant ipilimumab in comparison with placebo in patients with high-risk stage III disease. The trial excluded patients who had less than or equal to 1 mm lymph node and in transit metastases. Ipilimumab resulted in higher 5-year disease-free survival rates (40.8% vs 30.3% in the ipilimumab and placebo groups, respectively). Improved recurrence-free survival was transitioned to higher overall survival with a 5-year overall survival rate of 65% in the ipilimumab group. Ipilimumab resulted in grade 3 and higher toxicity in one-half of patients resulting to drug discontinuation.[119,120] Based on the results,

ipilimumab was approved by the FDA in 2015 as an adjuvant therapy for the management of patients with stage III disease who underwent wide local excision of primary tumor along with lymphadenectomy. The North American Intergroup trial E1609 further investigated the role of ipilimumab in the adjuvant setting, comparing ipilimumab at the dose of 3 mg/kg in relation to high-dose interferon, and ipilimumab at the dose of 10 mg/kg to high-dose interferon. Ipilimumab 3 mg/kg resulted in improved overall survival but not relapse-free survival in comparison with high-dose interferon. Ipilimumab 10 mg/kg did not improve relapse-free survival/overall survival and resulted in higher toxicity.[121]

Adjuvant anti–programmed death 1

Checkmate 238 compared 3 mg/kg nivolumab with 10 mg/kg ipilimumab as approved on the basis of EORTC 18071 in 2015, in the adjuvant setting. The trial excluded patients with stage IIIA disease and included patients with resected solitary stage IV melanoma. Nivolumab resulted in higher 1-year disease-free survival rate (71% vs 61% in the nivolumab and ipilimumab groups, respectively), and was better tolerated.[122] EORTC1325/Keynote 054 included patients with stage IIIA (>1 mm nodal disease burden), IIIB and IIIC, *BRAF* wild-type and mutated melanoma. Pembrolizumab improved disease-free survival in comparison with placebo, resulting in a 1-year relapse-free survival rate of 75.4%. The benefit was seen in both *BRAF* wild-type and *v600E* mutated cases. Pembrolizumab was well-tolerated in comparison with single agent ipilimumab and resulted in grade 3 and higher TRAEs in 14.7% of patients.[123] These trials resulted in FDA approval of nivolumab in 2017 and pembrolizumab in 2019. Based on safety and efficacy results, these are the preferred agents over ipilimumab and interferon. The Checkmate915 trial of BMS has reported no benefit from the combination of adjuvant ipilimumab and nivolumab in patients with stages III and IV resected disease with PD ligand 1 of less than 1%. The study remains blinded to evaluate the efficacy in the intention-to-treat population.

Adjuvant BRAFi or BRAFi/MEKi Oral Targeted Therapy

BRIM8 investigated the role of adjuvant vemurafenib in the adjuvant setting comparing it with placebo. This study included 2 cohorts separating patients with stage IIC, IIIA, and IIIB disease (cohort 1) and IIIC disease (cohort 2). Vemurafenib failed to show statistically improved relapse-free survival over placebo in patients with stage IIIC disease. In cohort 1, vemurafenib resulted in a 46% decrease in relapse-free survival; however, the result is not significant owing to prespecified hierarchical study design.[124] Single agent BRAF inhibitor was not approved by the FDA in the adjuvant setting.

Dabrafenib in combination with trametinib is the only *BRAF/MEK* inhibitor therapy that has been tested in a placebo-controlled prospective trial, with FDA approval in 2018 for adjuvant therapy. Dabrafenib in combination with trametinib is associated with improved relapse-free survival and overall survival in comparison with placebo, with a 3-year relapse-free survival rate of 58% in patients with *BRAFv600E/K* mutation–positive stage III melanoma.[125] The combination also resulted in clinically meaningful improvements in overall survival, decreasing the risk of death by 43%. Grade 3 and higher adverse events were reported in 41% patients, which was less than is noted for this regimen in the metastatic setting, although discontinuation rates were higher in the adjuvant compared with the metastatic setting (26% vs 15%, respectively). Adverse event rates decreased with increased time on treatment in both settings.[126]

Neoadjuvant Therapy

Despite major advancements in the adjuvant therapeutic options and improvement in relapse-free survival in patients with stage III, a significant fraction of patients still experience recurrent disease, raising the need to rapidly explore the multiple new options of targeted therapy and immunotherapy in the patients with melanoma. Therefore, the neoadjuvant setting was first explored in the context of a preoperative intervention of 1 month before definitive surgery, in which the preoperative setting also allowed the exploration of relevant mechanisms of action for biological agents like interferon. The goals of neoadjuvant therapy were also to decrease tumor burden and to improve the success of surgical management and decrease the morbidity associated with the procedure, to rapidly evaluate the objective clinical and radiologic responses to specific neoadjuvant therapy and guide further management in the adjuvant setting. The neoadjuvant approach provides an opportunity to monitor changes in the tumor microenvironment before and after treatment and to evaluate pathologic response to the treatment, which is considered as an end point in the neoadjuvant trials. There are not yet sufficient data to allow us to consider neoadjuvant therapy as a standard of care, but ongoing and completed phase I and II trials showed promising results. The main end point of neoadjuvant trials to date has been the pathologic response rate, which is defined as complete absence of viable tumor cells (pCR) or less than 10% of tumor remaining (pMR), along with the observed response rate judged before definitive surgery, and the usual parameters of relapse-free survival and overall survival.

In the early 2000s, the role of high-dose interferon was investigated in the neoadjuvant setting by our group. high-dose interferon had an immunomodulatory effect on tumor microenvironment resulting in increase in intratumoral CD11c$^+$ and CD3$^+$ cells and pathologic complete response rate of 15%. The toxicity resulted in drug discontinuation in one-fourth of patients.[127] High-dose ipilimumab resulted in favorable changes in the tumor microenvironment becoming a base to further explore checkpoint blockade therapy in the neoadjuvant settings.[128] However, high-dose (10 mg/kg) ipilimumab did not result in pathologic complete responses and 40% of patients had grade 3 toxicity. Neoadjuvant ipilimumab in combination with high-dose interferon resulted in pCR of 32%.[129] The combination of ipilimumab and nivolumab resulted in major pathologic response in 78% of patients.[130] As expected, the combination was associated with high toxicity G3 and higher adverse events reported in 90% of patients. The Opacin-neo trial did not include adjuvant treatment and compared different doses of ipilimumab and nivolumab combination to find safer and higher efficacious combination. Nivolumab at the dose of 3 mg/kg with ipilimumab at 1 g/kg was safe and associated with pCR of 57%.[131] Single-agent nivolumab resulted in pCR of 25%, but was well-tolerated in comparison with the combination of nivolumab and ipilimumab, which was associated with pCR of 45% and grade 3 and higher treatment-related adverse events of 78%.[132] A single dose of pembrolizumab resulted in pCR of 30%, and the pCR was correlated with disease-free survival.[133] Dabrafenib in combination with trametinib resulted in pCR of 58% and was well-tolerated.[134] It is important to note that, in a pooled analysis of targeted therapy and immunotherapy, pCR was correlated with disease-free survival with no relapse-free survival in patients treated with neoadjuvant immunotherapy and a 41% relapse-free survival rate after targeted therapy.[135] Even though BRAF/MEK inhibition can result in high pCR, the recurrence of disease can still present in contrast with immunotherapy. In summary, the role of neoadjuvant therapy is being actively explored in the management of resectable stage

III and IV disease. There is no randomized controlled trial comparing direct adjuvant and neoadjuvant approach for stage III patients. SWOG1801 is an ongoing randomized phase II trial comparing adjuvant versus both neoadjuvant and adjuvant pembrolizumab in resectable stage III to IV melanoma (NCT03698019). Although not being a standard of care approach for patients with melanoma, it is encouraging for patients to enroll in clinical trials to further expand the knowledge about the role of neoadjuvant therapy.

DISCUSSION AND FUTURE DIRECTIONS

Historically, melanoma has been considered as being one of highest mortality cancers without significant improvement for almost 35 years in the overall survival of patients. Continuous efforts of our group and others resulted in major advancements in the field. However, patients with brain metastases, elevated lactate dehydrogenase at baseline, and more than 3 metastatic sites continue to have a worse prognosis, raising the need for further advancements.

The standard of care for higher risk stage IIB and IIC and for stage IIIA disease remains an area in flux, where further investigations are currently in progress. The 5-year melanoma-specific survival for stage IIB and IIC disease (AJCC 8th ed) are 87% and 82%, respectively, and the pattern of relapse risk extends significantly past this window. The role of adjuvant pembrolizumab and nivolumab is currently being evaluated in phase III placebo-controlled trials.[136,137] The role of adjuvant therapy in stage IIIA melanoma, in comparison with observation, is an area of intense discussion, as many adjuvant trials have not included patients with less than 1 mm microscopic lymph node disease. Whether it is worth the risk of adverse events owing to immunotherapy for patients with a 5-year melanoma-specific survival of 93% is under exploration, but in young patients the horizon of 20 years may be more relevant to these considerations. The limited horizon for melanoma-specific survival in the 8th edition of the AJCC staging database is therefore one issue, because it is clearly recognized that disease-related events occur out to 20 years, and beyond. Neoadjuvant therapy is being actively explored in patients with stage IIIB and IIIC disease, but no head-to-head comparative trials are available to establish the benefit of the neoadjuvant approach over the standard postoperative adjuvant approach at this time.

In the era of available multiple therapeutic options, it remains an unanswered question whether BRAF/MEK targeted therapy or immunotherapy or the combination of BRAF/MEK with anti-PD1 therapy should be considered the first line of therapy in patients with BRAF-mutant cutaneous melanoma. The failure of the Keynote 022 and Combi-I trials to reach their primary goals are cautionary. In addition, the optimal sequence of immune checkpoint blockade and targeted therapy is not known either. The role of biomarkers beyond BRAF mutation in guiding adjuvant therapy or advanced disease therapy is an area of key importance, beyond the scope of this historic review.

ClinicalTrials.gov includes 62 recruiting interventional trials at this point for stage III and IV melanoma with the goal to further improve the outcome of patients with systemic disease, in particular those who progress on standard of care anti-PDA1/CTLA4 and BRAF/MEK inhibitor therapies. Different mechanistic approaches are being targeted, which include but are not limited to induction of innate immune response with Toll-like receptor, STING agonists, Radiation therapy, targeting inhibitory pathways with IDO and arginase inhibitors, angiogenesis inhibitors such as anti-vascular endothelial growth factor therapies, and other inhibitory receptors such as anti-LAG3 and anti-TIM3. The enrollment of patients in new clinical trials is to be encouraged to achieve the next milestones, of improved cure for patients with locoregionally advanced operable, as well as inoperable melanoma.

CLINICS CARE POINTS

- The management for Stage I/II melanoma includes wide local excision with proper surgical margins.
- Sentinel lymph node evaluation is indicated for proper staging.
- Anti-PD1 and Anti-CTLA4 and BRAF/MEK targeted therapies are two major therapeutic drugs for the management of advanced/unresectable melanoma.

ACKNOWLEDGMENTS

The authors thank Anca Tilea for her help with the preparation of figures.

DISCLOSURE

L. Karapetyan declares no disclosures or conflicts of interest. J.M. Kirkwood Consulting: Amgen, Inc., BMS, Checkmate, Novartis. Research support to institution: Amgen, BMS, Checkmate, Castle Biosciences, Inc., Immunocore LLC, Iovance, Novartis.

REFERENCES

1. Urteaga O, Pack GT. On the antiquity of melanoma. Cancer 1966;19(5):607–10.
2. Rebecca VW, Sondak VK, Smalley KSM. A brief history of melanoma: from mummies to mutations. Melanoma Res 2012;22(2):114–22.
3. Surveillance, Epidemiology, and End Results (SEER) Program Populations (1969-2018) (www.seer.cancer.gov/popdata), National Cancer Institute, DCCPS, Surveillance Research Program, released December 2019.
4. Siegel RL, Miller KD, Jemal A. Cancer statistics, 2020. CA Cancer J Clin 2020; 70(1):7–30.
5. Morton DL, Eilber FR, Joseph WL, et al. Immunological factors in human sarcomas and melanomas: a rational basis for immunotherapy. Ann Surg 1970; 172(4):740–9.
6. Morton DL, Malmgren RA, Holmes EC, et al. Demonstration of antibodies against human malignant melanoma by immunofluorescence. Surgery 1968; 64(1):233–40.
7. Sumner WC, Foraker AG. Spontaneous regression of human melanoma: clinical and experimental studies. Cancer 1960;13:79–81.
8. Morton DL, Eilber FR, Holmes EC, et al. BCG immunotherapy of malignant melanoma: summary of a seven-year experience. Ann Surg 1974;180(4):635–43.
9. Kirkwood JM, Ernstoff MS. Interferons in the treatment of human cancer. J Clin Oncol 1984;2(4):336–52.
10. Kirkwood JM, Ibrahim JG, Sondak VK, et al. High- and low-dose interferon alfa-2b in high-risk melanoma: first analysis of intergroup trial E1690/S9111/C9190. J Clin Oncol 2000;18(12):2444–58.
11. Kirkwood JM, Ibrahim JG, Sosman JA, et al. High-dose interferon alfa-2b significantly prolongs relapse-free and overall survival compared with the GM2-KLH/QS-21 vaccine in patients with resected stage IIB-III melanoma: results of intergroup trial E1694/S9512/C509801. J Clin Oncol 2001;19(9):2370–80.
12. Eggermont AM, Suciu S, Santinami M, et al. Adjuvant therapy with pegylated interferon alfa-2b versus observation alone in resected stage III melanoma: final

results of EORTC 18991, a randomised phase III trial. Lancet 2008;372(9633): 117–26.

13. Morgan D, Ruscetti F, Gallo R. Selective in vitro growth of T lymphocytes from normal human bone marrows. Science 1976;193(4257):1007–8.

14. Atkins MB, Lotze MT, Dutcher JP, et al. High-dose recombinant interleukin 2 therapy for patients with metastatic melanoma: analysis of 270 patients treated between 1985 and 1993. J Clin Oncol 1999;17(7):2105.

15. Atkins MB, Kunkel L, Sznol M, et al. High-dose recombinant interleukin-2 therapy in patients with metastatic melanoma: long-term survival update. Cancer J Sci Am 2000;6(Suppl 1):S11–4.

16. Ives NJ, Stowe RL, Lorigan P, et al. Chemotherapy compared with biochemotherapy for the treatment of metastatic melanoma: a meta-analysis of 18 trials involving 2,621 patients. J Clin Oncol 2007;25(34):5426–34.

17. Testori A, Richards J, Whitman E, et al. Phase III comparison of vitespen, an autologous tumor-derived heat shock protein gp96 peptide complex vaccine, with physician's choice of treatment for stage IV melanoma: the C-100-21 Study Group. J Clin Oncol 2008;26(6):955–62.

18. Eggermont AMM, Suciu S, Rutkowski P, et al. Adjuvant ganglioside GM2-KLH/QS-21 vaccination versus observation after resection of primary tumor > 1.5 mm in patients with stage II melanoma: results of the EORTC 18961 randomized phase III trial. J Clin Oncol 2013;31(30):3831–7.

19. Sondak VK, Liu PY, Tuthill RJ, et al. Adjuvant immunotherapy of resected, intermediate-thickness, node-negative melanoma with an allogeneic tumor vaccine: overall results of a randomized trial of the Southwest Oncology Group. J Clin Oncol 2002;20(8):2058–66.

20. Morton DL, Foshag LJ, Hoon DS, et al. Prolongation of survival in metastatic melanoma after active specific immunotherapy with a new polyvalent melanoma vaccine. Ann Surg 1992;216(4):463–82.

21. Morton DL, Mozzillo N, Thompson JF, et al. An international, randomized, phase III trial of bacillus Calmette-Guerin (BCG) plus allogeneic melanoma vaccine (MCV) or placebo after complete resection of melanoma metastatic to regional or distant sites. J Clin Oncol 2007;25(18_suppl):8508.

22. Slingluff CLJ. The present and future of peptide vaccines for cancer: single or multiple, long or short, alone or in combination? Cancer J 2011;17(5):343–50.

23. Ozao-Choy J, Lee DJ, Faries MB. Melanoma vaccines: mixed past, promising future. Surg Clin North Am 2014;94(5):1017–30, viii.

24. Schwartzentruber DJ, Lawson DH, Richards JM, et al. gp100 Peptide Vaccine and Interleukin-2 in Patients with Advanced Melanoma. N Engl J Med 2011; 364(22):2119–27.

25. Saiag P, Gutzmer R, Ascierto PA, et al. Prospective assessment of a gene signature potentially predictive of clinical benefit in metastatic melanoma patients following MAGE-A3 immunotherapeutic (PREDICT). Ann Oncol 2016;27(10): 1947–53.

26. Lipson EJ, Sharfman WH, Chen S, et al. Safety and immunologic correlates of Melanoma GVAX, a GM-CSF secreting allogeneic melanoma cell vaccine administered in the adjuvant setting. J Transl Med 2015;13:214.

27. Leach DR, Krummel MF, Allison JP. Enhancement of Antitumor Immunity by CTLA-4 Blockade. Science 1996;271(5256):1734–6.

28. Norris W. Eight cases of Melanosis with pathological and therapeutical remarks on that disease. London: Longman; 1857.

29. Cooper S. The First Lines of the Theory and Practice of Surgery. London: Longman; 1840.
30. Veronesi U, Cascinelli N. Narrow excision (1-cm margin). A safe procedure for thin cutaneous melanoma. Arch Surg 1991;126(4):438–41.
31. Veronesi U, Cascinelli N, Adamus J, et al. Thin stage I primary cutaneous malignant melanoma. Comparison of excision with margins of 1 or 3 cm. N Engl J Med 1988;318(18):1159–62.
32. Cohn-Cedermark G, Rutqvist LE, Andersson R, et al. Long term results of a randomized study by the Swedish Melanoma Study Group on 2-cm versus 5-cm resection margins for patients with cutaneous melanoma with a tumor thickness of 0.8-2.0 mm. Cancer 2000;89(7):1495–501.
33. Khayat D, Rixe O, Martin G, et al. Surgical margins in cutaneous melanoma (2 cm versus 5 cm for lesions measuring less than 2.1-mm thick). Cancer 2003;97(8):1941–6.
34. Balch CM, Soong SJ, Smith T, et al. Long-term results of a prospective surgical trial comparing 2 cm vs. 4 cm excision margins for 740 patients with 1-4 mm melanomas. Ann Surg Oncol 2001;8(2):101–8.
35. Gillgren P, Drzewiecki KT, Niin M, et al. 2-cm versus 4-cm surgical excision margins for primary cutaneous melanoma thicker than 2 mm: a randomised, multicentre trial. Lancet 2011;378(9803):1635–42.
36. Hayes AJ, Maynard L, Coombes G, et al. Wide versus narrow excision margins for high-risk, primary cutaneous melanomas: long-term follow-up of survival in a randomised trial. Lancet Oncol 2016;17(2):184–92.
37. Thomas JM, Newton-Bishop J, A'Hern R, et al. Excision margins in high-risk malignant melanoma. N Engl J Med 2004;350(8):757–66.
38. Lee MP, Sobanko JF, Shin TM, et al. Evolution of Excisional Surgery Practices for Melanoma in the United States. JAMA Dermatol 2019;155(11):1244–51.
39. Cheraghlou S, Christensen SR, Agogo GO, et al. Comparison of survival after Mohs micrographic surgery vs wide margin excision for early-stage invasive melanoma. JAMA Dermatol 2019;155(11):1252–9.
40. Neuhaus SJ, Clark MA, Thomas JM. Dr. Herbert Lumley Snow, MD, MRCS (1847-1930): the original champion of elective lymph node dissection in melanoma. Ann Surg Oncol 2004;11(9):875–8.
41. Cascinelli N, Morabito A, Santinami M, et al. Immediate or delayed dissection of regional nodes in patients with melanoma of the trunk: a randomised trial. Lancet 1998;351(9105):793–6.
42. Morton DL, Wen DR, Wong JH, et al. Technical details of intraoperative lymphatic mapping for early stage melanoma. Arch Surg 1992;127(4):392–9.
43. Cordeiro E, Gervais M-K, Shah PS, et al. Sentinel lymph node biopsy in thin cutaneous melanoma: a systematic review and meta-analysis. Ann Surg Oncol 2016;23(13):4178–88.
44. Gershenwald JE, Scolyer RA, Hess KR, et al. Melanoma staging: evidence-based changes in the American Joint Committee on Cancer eighth edition cancer staging manual. CA Cancer J Clin 2017;67(6):472–92.
45. Lo SN, Ma J, Scolyer RA, et al. Improved risk prediction calculator for sentinel node positivity in patients with melanoma: the Melanoma Institute Australia Nomogram. J Clin Oncol 2020;19:02362.
46. Gershenwald JE, Thompson W, Mansfield PF, et al. Multi-institutional melanoma lymphatic mapping experience: the prognostic value of sentinel lymph node status in 612 stage I or II melanoma patients. J Clin Oncol 1999;17(3):976–83.

47. Morton DL, Thompson JF, Cochran AJ, et al. Sentinel-Node Biopsy or Nodal Observation in Melanoma. N Engl J Med 2006;355(13):1307–17.

48. Theodore JE, Frankel AJ, Thomas JM, et al. Assessment of morbidity following regional nodal dissection in the axilla and groin for metastatic melanoma. ANZ J Surg 2017;87(1–2):44–8.

49. Guggenheim MM, Hug U, Jung FJ, et al. Morbidity and recurrence after completion lymph node dissection following sentinel lymph node biopsy in cutaneous malignant melanoma. Ann Surg 2008;247(4):687–93.

50. Faries MB, Thompson JF, Cochran AJ, et al. Completion Dissection or Observation for Sentinel-Node Metastasis in Melanoma. N Engl J Med 2017;376(23): 2211–22.

51. Leiter U, Stadler R, Mauch C, et al. Final analysis of DeCOG-SLT trial: no survival benefit for complete lymph node dissection in patients with melanoma with positive sentinel node. J Clin Oncol 2019;37(32):3000–8.

52. Glover AR, Allan CP, Wilkinson MJ, et al. Outcomes of routine ilioinguinal lymph node dissection for palpable inguinal melanoma nodal metastasis. Br J Surg 2014;101(7):811–9.

53. Kretschmer L, Neumann C, Preusser KP, et al. Superficial inguinal and radical ilioinguinal lymph node dissection in patients with palpable melanoma metastases to the groin–an analysis of survival and local recurrence. Acta Oncol 2001; 40(1):72–8.

54. Balch CM, Gershenwald JE, Soong S-J, et al. Final version of 2009 AJCC melanoma staging and classification. J Clin Oncol 2009;27(36):6199–206.

55. Andtbacka RHI, Kaufman HL, Collichio F, et al. Talimogene laherparepvec improves durable response rate in patients with advanced melanoma. J Clin Oncol 2015;33(25):2780–8.

56. Larkin J, Chiarion-Sileni V, Gonzalez R, et al. Five-year survival with combined nivolumab and ipilimumab in advanced melanoma. N Engl J Med 2019; 381(16):1535–46.

57. Robert C, Grob JJ, Stroyakovskiy D, et al. Five-year outcomes with dabrafenib plus trametinib in metastatic melanoma. N Engl J Med 2019;381(7):626–36.

58. Patel PM, Suciu S, Mortier L, et al. Extended schedule, escalated dose temozolomide versus dacarbazine in stage IV melanoma: final results of a randomised phase III study (EORTC 18032). Eur J Cancer 2011;47(10):1476–83.

59. Costanza ME, Nathanson L, Lenhard R, et al. Therapy of malignant melanoma with an imidazole carboxamide and bis-chloroethyl nitrosourea. Cancer 1972; 30(6):1457–61.

60. Hill GJ 2nd, Krementz ET, Hill HZ. Dimethyl triazeno imidazole carboxamide and combination therapy for melanoma. IV. Late results after complete response to chemotherapy (Central Oncology Group protocols 7130, 7131, and 7131A). Cancer 1984;53(6):1299–305.

61. Lui P, Cashin R, Machado M, et al. Treatments for metastatic melanoma: synthesis of evidence from randomized trials. Cancer Treat Rev 2007;33(8):665–80.

62. Chapman PB, Einhorn LH, Meyers ML, et al. Phase III multicenter randomized trial of the Dartmouth regimen versus dacarbazine in patients with metastatic melanoma. J Clin Oncol 1999;17(9):2745–51.

63. Hersh EM, Del Vecchio M, Brown MP, et al. A randomized, controlled phase III trial of nab-Paclitaxel versus dacarbazine in chemotherapy-naïve patients with metastatic melanoma. Ann Oncol 2015;26(11):2267–74.

64. Kirkwood JM, Strawderman MH, Ernstoff MS, et al. Interferon alfa-2b adjuvant therapy of high-risk resected cutaneous melanoma: the Eastern Cooperative Oncology Group Trial EST 1684. J Clin Oncol 1996;14(1):7–17.

65. Livingston PO, Wong GY, Adluri S, et al. Improved survival in stage III melanoma patients with GM2 antibodies: a randomized trial of adjuvant vaccination with GM2 ganglioside. J Clin Oncol 1994;12(5):1036–44.

66. McMasters KM, Egger ME, Edwards MJ, et al. Final results of the sunbelt melanoma trial: a multi-institutional prospective randomized phase iii study evaluating the role of adjuvant high-dose interferon alfa-2b and completion lymph node dissection for patients staged by sentinel lymph node biopsy. J Clin Oncol 2016;34(10):1079–86.

67. Agarwala SS, Lee SJ, Yip W, et al. Phase III randomized study of 4 weeks of high-dose interferon-α-2b in stage T2bNO, T3a-bNO, T4a-bNO, and T1-4N1a-2a (microscopic) melanoma: a trial of the Eastern Cooperative Oncology Group–American College of Radiology Imaging Network Cancer Research Group (E1697). J Clin Oncol 2017;35(8):885–92.

68. Hansson J, Aamdal S, Bastholt L, et al. Two different durations of adjuvant therapy with intermediate-dose interferon alfa-2b in patients with high-risk melanoma (Nordic IFN trial): a randomised phase 3 trial. Lancet Oncol 2011;12(2):144–52.

69. Suciu S, Eggermont AMM, Lorigan P, et al. Relapse-free survival as a surrogate for overall survival in the evaluation of stage II-III melanoma adjuvant therapy. J Natl Cancer Inst 2018;110(1). https://doi.org/10.1093/jnci/djx133.

70. Jonasch E, Haluska FG. Interferon in oncological practice: review of interferon biology, clinical applications, and toxicities. Oncologist 2001;6(1):34–55.

71. Gogas H, Ioannovich J, Dafni U, et al. Prognostic significance of autoimmunity during treatment of melanoma with interferon. N Engl J Med 2006;354(7):709–18.

72. Seth R, Messersmith H, Kaur V, et al. Systemic therapy for melanoma: ASCO guideline. J Clin Oncol 2020. https://doi.org/10.1200/JCO.20.00198.

73. Lotze MT, Grimm EA, Mazumder A, et al. Lysis of fresh and cultured autologous tumor by human lymphocytes cultured in T-cell growth factor. Cancer Res 1981;41(11 Pt 1):4420–5.

74. Rosenberg SA, Lotze MT, Muul LM, et al. Observations on the systemic administration of autologous lymphokine-activated killer cells and recombinant interleukin-2 to patients with metastatic cancer. N Engl J Med 1985;313(23):1485–92.

75. Lotze MT, Matory YL, Rayner AA, et al. Clinical effects and toxicity of interleukin-2 in patients with cancer. Cancer 1986;58(12):2764–72.

76. White RL Jr, Schwartzentruber DJ, Guleria A, et al. Cardiopulmonary toxicity of treatment with high dose interleukin-2 in 199 consecutive patients with metastatic melanoma or renal cell carcinoma. Cancer 1994;74(12):3212–22.

77. Guleria AS, Yang JC, Topalian SL, et al. Renal dysfunction associated with the administration of high-dose interleukin-2 in 199 consecutive patients with metastatic melanoma or renal carcinoma. J Clin Oncol 1994;12(12):2714–22.

78. MacFarlane MP, Yang JC, Guleria AS, et al. The hematologic toxicity of interleukin-2 in patients with metastatic melanoma and renal cell carcinoma. Cancer 1995;75(4):1030–7.

79. Kammula US, White DE, Rosenberg SA. Trends in the safety of high dose bolus interleukin-2 administration in patients with metastatic cancer. Cancer 1998;83(4):797–805.

80. Byers BA, Temple-Oberle CF, Hurdle V, et al. Treatment of in-transit melanoma with intra-lesional interleukin-2: a systematic review. J Surg Oncol 2014; 110(6):770–5.
81. Hodi FS, O'Day SJ, McDermott DF, et al. Improved survival with ipilimumab in patients with metastatic melanoma. N Engl J Med 2010;363(8):711–23.
82. Robert C, Thomas L, Bondarenko I, et al. Ipilimumab plus dacarbazine for previously untreated metastatic melanoma. N Engl J Med 2011;364(26):2517–26.
83. Hodi FS, Lee S, McDermott DF, et al. Ipilimumab plus sargramostim vs ipilimumab alone for treatment of metastatic melanoma: a randomized clinical trial. JAMA 2014;312(17):1744–53.
84. Ascierto PA, Del Vecchio M, Robert C, et al. Ipilimumab 10 mg/kg versus ipilimumab 3 mg/kg in patients with unresectable or metastatic melanoma: a randomised, double-blind, multicentre, phase 3 trial. Lancet Oncol 2017;18(5): 611–22.
85. Ribas A, Kefford R, Marshall MA, et al. Phase III randomized clinical trial comparing tremelimumab with standard-of-care chemotherapy in patients with advanced melanoma. J Clin Oncol 2013;31(5):616–22.
86. Robert C, Long GV, Brady B, et al. Nivolumab in previously untreated melanoma without BRAF mutation. N Engl J Med 2014;372(4):320–30.
87. Weber JS, D'Angelo SP, Minor D, et al. Nivolumab versus chemotherapy in patients with advanced melanoma who progressed after anti-CTLA-4 treatment (CheckMate 037): a randomised, controlled, open-label, phase 3 trial. Lancet Oncol 2015;16(4):375–84.
88. Robert C, Schachter J, Long GV, et al. Pembrolizumab versus Ipilimumab in Advanced Melanoma. N Engl J Med 2015;372(26):2521–32.
89. Long GV, Schachter J, Ribas A, et al. 4-year survival and outcomes after cessation of pembrolizumab (pembro) after 2-years in patients (pts) with ipilimumab (ipi)-naive advanced melanoma in KEYNOTE-006. J Clin Oncol 2018; 36(15_suppl):9503.
90. Puzanov I, Ribas A, Robert C, et al. Association of BRAF V600E/K Mutation Status and Prior BRAF/MEK inhibition with pembrolizumab outcomes in advanced melanoma: pooled analysis of 3 clinical trials. JAMA Oncol 2020;6(8):1256–64.
91. Larkin J, Chiarion-Sileni V, Gonzalez R, et al. Combined nivolumab and ipilimumab or monotherapy in untreated melanoma. N Engl J Med 2015;373(1):23–34.
92. Lebbé C, Meyer N, Mortier L, et al. Evaluation of two dosing regimens for nivolumab in combination with ipilimumab in patients with advanced melanoma: results from the phase IIIb/IV CheckMate 511 Trial. J Clin Oncol 2019;37(11): 867–75.
93. Davies MA, Liu P, McIntyre S, et al. Prognostic factors for survival in melanoma patients with brain metastases. Cancer 2011;117(8):1687–96.
94. Tawbi HA-H, Forsyth PAJ, Hodi FS, et al. Efficacy and safety of the combination of nivolumab (NIVO) plus ipilimumab (IPI) in patients with symptomatic melanoma brain metastases (CheckMate 204). J Clin Oncol 2019;37(15_suppl): 9501.
95. Tawbi HA, Forsyth PA, Algazi A, et al. Combined nivolumab and ipilimumab in melanoma metastatic to the brain. N Engl J Med 2018;379(8):722–30.
96. Daniel Olson JJL, Andrew Stewart P, Madhuri B, et al. Significant antitumor activity for low-dose ipilimumab (IPI) with pembrolizumab (PEMBRO) immediately following progression on PD1 Ab in melanoma (MEL) in a phase II trial. J Clin Oncol 2020;38:2020.

97. Omholt K, Platz A, Kanter L, et al. NRAS and BRAF mutations arise early during melanoma pathogenesis and are preserved throughout tumor progression. Clin Cancer Res 2003;9(17):6483–8.
98. Davies H, Bignell GR, Cox C, et al. Mutations of the BRAF gene in human cancer. Nature 2002;417(6892):949–54.
99. Cancer Genome Atlas Network. Genomic classification of cutaneous melanoma. Cell 2015;161(7):1681–96.
100. Flaherty KT, Lee SJ, Zhao F, et al. Phase III trial of carboplatin and paclitaxel with or without sorafenib in metastatic melanoma. J Clin Oncol 2013;31(3):373–9.
101. Flaherty KT, Schiller J, Schuchter LM, et al. A Phase I trial of the oral, multikinase inhibitor sorafenib in combination with carboplatin and paclitaxel. Clin Cancer Res 2008;14(15):4836–42.
102. Sosman JA, Kim KB, Schuchter L, et al. Survival in BRAF V600–mutant advanced melanoma treated with vemurafenib. N Engl J Med 2012;366(8):707–14.
103. Chapman PB, Hauschild A, Robert C, et al. Improved Survival with Vemurafenib in Melanoma with BRAF V600E Mutation. N Engl J Med 2011;364(26):2507–16.
104. Hauschild A, Grob J-J, Demidov LV, et al. Dabrafenib in BRAF-mutated metastatic melanoma: a multicentre, open-label, phase 3 randomised controlled trial. Lancet 2012;380(9839):358–65.
105. Flaherty KT, Robert C, Hersey P, et al. Improved Survival with MEK Inhibition in BRAF-Mutated Melanoma. N Engl J Med 2012;367(2):107–14.
106. Long GV, Stroyakovskiy D, Gogas H, et al. Combined BRAF and MEK Inhibition versus BRAF inhibition alone in melanoma. N Engl J Med 2014;371(20):1877–88.
107. Long GV, Stroyakovskiy D, Gogas H, et al. Dabrafenib and trametinib versus dabrafenib and placebo for Val600 BRAF-mutant melanoma: a multicentre, double-blind, phase 3 randomised controlled trial. Lancet 2015;386(9992):444–51.
108. Robert C, Karaszewska B, Schachter J, et al. Improved overall survival in melanoma with combined dabrafenib and trametinib. N Engl J Med 2014;372(1):30–9.
109. Long GV, Grob J-J, Nathan P, et al. Factors predictive of response, disease progression, and overall survival after dabrafenib and trametinib combination treatment: a pooled analysis of individual patient data from randomised trials. Lancet Oncol 2016;17(12):1743–54.
110. Larkin J, Ascierto PA, Dréno B, et al. Combined vemurafenib and cobimetinib in BRAF-mutated melanoma. N Engl J Med 2014;371(20):1867–76.
111. McArthur GA DB, Larkin J, et al. 5-year survival update of cobimetinib plus vemurafenib BRAF V600 mutation-positive advanced melanoma: final analysis of the coBRIM study. Presented at: the 16th International Congress of the Society for Melanoma Research; November 20–23, 2019; Salt Lake City, UT.
112. Dummer R, Ascierto PA, Gogas HJ, et al. Encorafenib plus binimetinib versus vemurafenib or encorafenib in patients with BRAF-mutant melanoma (COLUMBUS): a multicentre, open-label, randomised phase 3 trial. Lancet Oncol 2018;19(5):603–15.
113. Dummer R, Ascierto PA, Gogas H, et al. Results of COLUMBUS part 2: a phase 3 trial of encorafenib (ENCO) plus binimetinib (BINI) versus ENCO in BRAF-mutant melanoma. Ann Oncol 2017;28(suppl 5):1215OA.
114. Frederick DT, Piris A, Cogdill AP, et al. BRAF inhibition is associated with enhanced melanoma antigen expression and a more favorable tumor

microenvironment in patients with metastatic melanoma. Clin Cancer Res 2013; 19(5):1225–31.

115. Cooper ZA, Juneja VR, Sage PT, et al. Response to BRAF inhibition in melanoma is enhanced when combined with immune checkpoint blockade. Cancer Immunol Res 2014;2(7):643–54.

116. McArthur GA, Stroyakovskiy D, Gogas H, et al. CT012 — Evaluation of atezolizumab (A), cobimetinib (C), and vemurafenib (V) in previously untreated patients with BRAFV600 mutation-positive advanced melanoma: primary results from the phase 3 IMspire150 trial. Presented at: the 2020 AACR Annual Virtual Meeting I; April 27–28, 2020 Abstract CT012. 2020.

117. Gutzmer R, Stroyakovskiy D, Gogas H, et al. Atezolizumab, vemurafenib, and cobimetinib as first-line treatment for unresectable advanced BRAFV600 mutation-positive melanoma (IMspire150): primary analysis of the randomised, double-blind, placebo-controlled, phase 3 trial. Lancet 2020;395(10240): 1835–44.

118. Long GV, Lebbe C, Atkinson V, et al. The anti–PD-1 antibody spartalizumab (S) in combination with dabrafenib (D) and trametinib (T) in previously untreated patients (pts) with advanced BRAF V600–mutant melanoma: updated efficacy and safety from parts 1 and 2 of COMBI-i. J Clin Oncol 2019;37(15_suppl):9531.

119. Eggermont AM, Chiarion-Sileni V, Grob JJ, et al. Prolonged survival in stage III melanoma with ipilimumab adjuvant therapy. N Engl J Med 2016;375(19): 1845–55.

120. Eggermont AM, Chiarion-Sileni V, Grob JJ, et al. Adjuvant ipilimumab versus placebo after complete resection of high-risk stage III melanoma (EORTC 18071): a randomised, double-blind, phase 3 trial. Lancet Oncol 2015;16(5): 522–30.

121. Tarhini AA, Lee SJ, Hodi FS, et al. Phase III study of adjuvant ipilimumab (3 or 10 mg/kg) versus high-dose interferon Alfa-2b for resected high-risk melanoma: North American Intergroup E1609. J Clin Oncol 2020;38(6):567–75.

122. Weber J, Mandala M, Del Vecchio M, et al. Adjuvant Nivolumab versus Ipilimumab in Resected Stage III or IV Melanoma. N Engl J Med 2017;377(19): 1824–35.

123. Eggermont AMM, Blank CU, Mandala M, et al. Adjuvant pembrolizumab versus placebo in resected stage III melanoma. N Engl J Med 2018;378(19):1789–801.

124. Maio M, Lewis K, Demidov L, et al. Adjuvant vemurafenib in resected, -BRAFV600 mutation-positive melanoma (BRIM8): a randomised, double-blind, placebo-controlled, multicentre, phase 3 trial. Lancet Oncol 2018;19(4): 510–20.

125. Long GV, Hauschild A, Santinami M, et al. Adjuvant Dabrafenib plus Trametinib in Stage III BRAF-Mutated Melanoma. N Engl J Med 2017;377(19):1813–23.

126. Grob JJ, Atkinson VG, Robert C, et al. 1333P - Adverse event (AE) kinetics in patients (pts) treated with dabrafenib + trametinib (D + T) in the metastatic and adjuvant setting. Ann Oncol 2019;30:v543–4.

127. Moschos SJ, Edington HD, Land SR, et al. Neoadjuvant Treatment of Regional Stage IIIB Melanoma With High-Dose Interferon Alfa-2b Induces Objective Tumor Regression in Association With Modulation of Tumor Infiltrating Host Cellular Immune Responses. J Clin Oncol 2006;24(19):3164–71.

128. Tarhini AA, Edington H, Butterfield LH, et al. Immune monitoring of the circulation and the tumor microenvironment in patients with regionally advanced melanoma receiving neoadjuvant ipilimumab. PLoS One 2014;9(2):e87705.

129. Tarhini A, Lin Y, Lin H, et al. Neoadjuvant ipilimumab (3 mg/kg or 10 mg/kg) and high dose IFN-α2b in locally/regionally advanced melanoma: safety, efficacy and impact on T-cell repertoire. J Immunother Cancer 2018;6(1):112.
130. Blank CU, Rozeman EA, Fanchi LF, et al. Neoadjuvant versus adjuvant ipilimumab plus nivolumab in macroscopic stage III melanoma. Nat Med 2018;24(11): 1655–61.
131. Rozeman EA, Menzies AM, van Akkooi ACJ, et al. Identification of the optimal combination dosing schedule of neoadjuvant ipilimumab plus nivolumab in macroscopic stage III melanoma (OpACIN-neo): a multicentre, phase 2, randomised, controlled trial. Lancet Oncol 2019;20(7):948–60.
132. Amaria RN, Reddy SM, Tawbi HA, et al. Neoadjuvant immune checkpoint blockade in high-risk resectable melanoma. Nat Med 2018;24(11):1649–54.
133. Huang AC, Orlowski RJ, Xu X, et al. A single dose of neoadjuvant PD-1 blockade predicts clinical outcomes in resectable melanoma. Nat Med 2019; 25(3):454–61.
134. Amaria RN, Prieto PA, Tetzlaff MT, et al. Neoadjuvant plus adjuvant dabrafenib and trametinib versus standard of care in patients with high-risk, surgically resectable melanoma: a single-centre, open-label, randomised, phase 2 trial. Lancet Oncol 2018;19(2):181–93.
135. Menzies AM, Rozeman EA, Amaria RN, et al. Pathological response and survival with neoadjuvant therapy in melanoma: a pooled analysis from the International Neoadjuvant Melanoma Consortium (INMC). J Clin Oncol 2019;37(15_suppl): 9503.
136. Luke JJ, Ascierto PA, Carlino MS, et al. KEYNOTE-716: phase III study of adjuvant pembrolizumab versus placebo in resected high-risk stage II melanoma. Future Oncol 2020;16(3):4429–38.
137. Poklepovic AS, Luke JJ. Considering adjuvant therapy for stage II melanoma. Cancer 2020;126(6):1166–74.
138. Gogas HJ, Kirkwood JM, Sondak VK. Chemotherapy for metastatic melanoma. Cancer 2007;109(3):455–64.
139. Larkin J, Minor D, D'Angelo S, et al. Overall survival in patients with advanced melanoma who received nivolumab versus investigator's choice chemotherapy in CheckMate 037: a randomized, controlled, open-label phase III trial. J Clin Oncol 2018;36(4):383–90.
140. Flaherty KT, Infante JR, Daud A, et al. Combined BRAF and MEK Inhibition in Melanoma with BRAF V600 Mutations. N Engl J Med 2012;367(18):1694–703.

Biology of Melanoma

Stephen M. Ostrowski, MD, PhD, David E. Fisher, MD, PhD*

KEYWORDS

• Melanocyte • Melanoma • MAPK • MITF • AXL • Immunotherapy

KEY POINTS

• Melanoma is the third commonest form of skin cancer, is derived from skin melanocytes, and has a high clinical impact because of early metastatic risk and poor prognosis of metastatic disease.
• The microphthalmia (MITF) transcription factor plays a central role in melanocyte and melanoma biology.
• The mitogen-activated protein kinase (MAPK) pathway plays a central role in melanogenesis, but clinical benefit of targeted inhibitors of BRAF and MEK are limited by near-universal development of resistance.
• Immunotherapy has transformed the treatment of metastatic melanoma, but innate and acquired resistance are common.
• Genetic mechanisms of resistance to therapy are common in melanoma. However, phenotypic plasticity that allows the development of the MITF^{low}/dedifferentiated cell state is a frequent mechanism of resistance to targeted therapy and immunotherapy.

INTRODUCTION

Melanoma skin cancer is derived from skin melanocytes and has a high risk of metastatic spread. Many clinical attributes and risk factors associated with melanoma have been well defined. The era of molecular genetics and next-generation sequencing has uncovered the role of oncogenic BRAF^{V600E} mutations in many melanomas, validated the role of ultraviolet (UV)-induced DNA mutations in melanoma formation, and uncovered many of the molecular events that occur during melanoma development. Targeted therapies and immunotherapy have dramatically improved outcomes and provided an increased rate of cure for metastatic melanoma. However, challenges remain in unraveling the biology of therapeutic resistance and relapse, which commonly occur. This article reviews the formation of melanoma from skin melanocytes, the molecular events involved in melanoma growth and metastasis, and the biology underlying resistance to melanoma therapies.

Department of Dermatology, Massachusetts General Hospital, Harvard Medical School, Bartlett 6, 55 Fruit Street, Boston, MA 02114, USA
* Corresponding author.
E-mail address: dfisher3@partners.org

Hematol Oncol Clin N Am 35 (2021) 29–56
https://doi.org/10.1016/j.hoc.2020.08.010
0889-8588/21/© 2020 Elsevier Inc. All rights reserved.

FROM MELANOCYTE TO MELANOMA
Melanocyte Biology and Nevus Formation

Melanocytes are neural crest-derived cells that exist primarily at the basal layer of the epidermis of human skin but are also located at other sites, including the hair follicle, uvea, mucosal epithelia, and meninges (**Fig. 1**). The primary function of cutaneous melanocytes is to synthesize melanin within organelles termed melanosomes, which are then transferred via dendritic processes to neighboring keratinocytes.[1–3] Within keratinocytes, melanosomes are localized to the perinuclear areas (nuclear capping) where they protect DNA from UV-mediated damage.[4] Melanogenesis and skin pigmentation are regulated by constitutive and adaptive pigmentation. Constitutive pigmentation represents the baseline level of skin pigmentation; this varies between different ethnic groups, and several genetic polymorphisms in key melanocyte signaling and pigment synthesis genes underlie many of these differences.[5] The best example of adaptive pigmentation is UV radiation–induced pigmentation (sun tanning), but this process can also become activated in disorders of skin hyperpigmentation.

Melanocytes produce two forms of melanin pigment, black/brown eumelanin and red/blond pheomelanin, which are both derived from the precursor tyrosine.[6] The balance between eumelanin and pheomelanin is regulated by signaling through the G

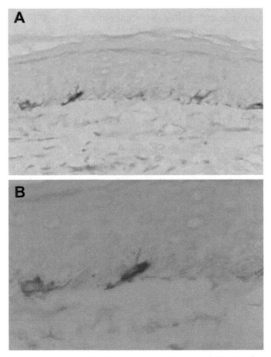

Fig. 1. Melanocytes are dendritic cells that exist at the basal layer of epidermis in interfollicular human skin. (*A*) Immunohistochemistry using antibody directed against Melan-A identifies melanocytes admixed with keratinocytes in the basal layer of epidermis (20X magnification). (*B*) Higher-power magnification shows the dendritic morphology of melanocytes (40X magnification). (*Courtesy of* Roberto Novoa MD, Stanford, CA.)

protein–coupled melanocortin-1 receptor (MC1R).[7] MC1R-dependent regulation of melanin synthesis in the UV-induced tanning pathway has been well characterized.[8] UV radiation leads to DNA damage within keratinocytes and subsequent p53 stabilization and direct transcriptional activation of proopiomelanocortin (POMC), which is posttranslationally processed into several peptides, including α-melanocyte–stimulating hormone (α-MSH).[8,9] α-MSH binds to and activates MC1R on the cell surface of melanocytes, leading to a cascade of activation of cyclic adenosine monophosphate (cAMP) and subsequent cAMP response element–binding protein (CREB)–mediated transcriptional activation of the transcription factor microphthalmia (MITF) (**Fig. 2**). It has also recently been appreciated that salt-inducible kinase (SIK) phosphorylation of CREB regulated transcription coactivator (CRTC) regulates MITF expression.[10,11]

MITF serves as the master regulator of the melanin synthesis pathway through direct transcriptional regulation of melanogenic enzymes such as PMEL, tyrosinase, TRP1, and DCT.[12,13] MITF also regulates the expression of numerous other target

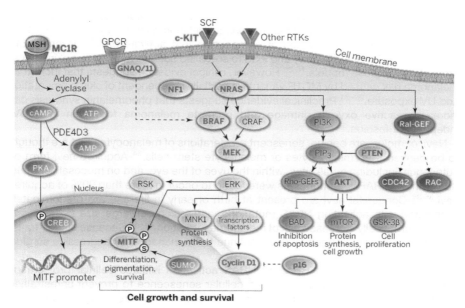

Fig. 2. Signaling pathways in melanocytes and melanoma. Mitogen-activated protein kinase (MAPK) signaling promotes cell growth and survival and is activated in most melanomas through activating mutation in BRAF or NRAS, or through inactivating mutation in neurofibromin 1 (NF1). KIT signaling is essential for melanocyte development and mutation and/or amplification of c-KIT is found in many melanomas arising on acral, mucosal, and chronically sun-damaged skin. Mutations in GNAQ and GNA11 are the main drivers of uveal melanomas. MITF acts as the master transcriptional regulator in melanocytes and also serves as a lineage oncogene. In melanocytes, MITF expression is regulated by MC1R signaling. Loss-of-function variants of MC1R are associated with the red hair/fair skin phenotype and increased melanoma susceptibility. Known melanoma oncogenes and tumor suppressors are labeled in red. Dotted lines represent omitted pathway components. (*From* Lo, J. A. & Fisher, D. E. The melanoma revolution: from UV carcinogenesis to a new era in therapeutics. *Science* 346, 945-949, https://doi.org/10.1126/science.1253735 (2014); with permission.)

genes that are important for the survival of melanocytes and melanoma cells, such as the antiapoptotic proteins BCL2 and BCL2A1, and the cell cycle regulator CDK2.[14–16] Hypomorphic mutation of MITF leads to Waardenburg syndrome type 2A in humans and severe loss-of-function mutation of MITF leads to complete absence of the melanocyte lineage in mice.[17,18] MITF is a sensitive and specific immunohistochemical marker in melanoma and is vital for survival of melanoma cells through lineage-specific regulation of the survival and antiapoptotic genes mentioned earlier.[15,16,19] Moreover, overactivity of MITF drives melanoma formation. This process is exemplified by oncogenic MITF amplifications in melanomas and oncogenic MITF dysregulation in clear cell sarcoma.[20,21] In addition, an activating mutation in MITF that modulates its transcriptional activity through disruption of a sumoylation consensus motif contributes to familial and sporadic melanoma formation in humans.[22,23]

Hypomorphic polymorphisms of MC1R are found frequently in northern European populations and these variants are largely responsible for red hair/fair skin/freckling phenotypes.[24] MC1R loss of function leads to decreased flux through the cAMP/PKA/SIK/MITF pathway and favors production of pheomelanin rather than eumelanin.[25] MC1R polymorphisms also dramatically increase melanoma risk and this may in part be caused by decreased protection from UV by pheomelanin, supported by increased UV signature mutational burdens in melanomas from patients with MC1R variants.[26,27] Topical application of compounds that activate cAMP or inhibit SIK can bypass MC1R insufficiency and lead to so-called sunless tanning and skin cancer prevention in mouse models.[10,28] However, clinical evidence suggests that increased melanoma risk caused by MC1R variants is partially independent of skin pigmentation and UV exposure.[29–31] Preclinical evidence suggests that pheomelanin synthesis can increase reactive oxygen damage and promote melanoma formation in a UV-independent fashion.[32,33]

Nevi, or moles, are benign, senescent proliferations of melanocytes that are thought to be derived from melanocytes or melanocyte stem cells.[34] Acquired nevi form on cutaneous (including acral) sites, within the uvea of the eye, and on mucosal surfaces. Surprisingly, BRAF^{V600E} mutations were found to occur in more than 90% of acquired nevi.[35,36] Congenital nevi are present at birth or early in life and are predominately associated with activating NRAS mutations, and lesions of large size (>20–40 cm) have a dramatically increased risk of melanoma formation.[37–40] Because of their transformation risk, giant congenital nevi continue to be managed by aggressive surgical resections.

It has been shown that BRAF or NRAS activation initiates cellular proliferation and nevus formation, but in turn drives cellular senescence to prevent unrestrained growth and malignant transformation.[34,41] Senescent nevi are benign lesions that show low numbers of mutations and copy number alterations compared with melanomas.[42–44] However, benign nevi can infrequently progress to melanoma.[45] Elegant studies by Shain and colleagues[46,47] confirmed a linear order of progression from precursor to melanoma and characterized the chronologic order of molecular events that occur in transition from benign nevus to melanoma in situ (MIS) to invasive melanoma. Briefly, early events (nevus to MIS) include increased mutational load, telomerase reverse transcriptase (TERT) promoter mutation, mutation of components of the SWI/SNF chromatin remodeling complex, and CDKN2A loss, whereas later events (progression from MIS to invasive melanoma) include copy number alterations and mutations in the p53 and phosphatase and tensin homologue (PTEN) pathways.[46,47] These molecular aberrations represent potential therapeutic targets, either directly (if druggable) or indirectly (through synthetic lethality).

Importantly, many studies suggest that only about 25% to 30% of melanomas are associated with a recognizable benign nevus precursor.[48] Members of melanoma-prone families were first noted to have clinically atypical moles that correlated with histologic dysplasia suggestive of precancerous changes (dysplastic nevi). It is generally well accepted that dysplastic nevi are common, benign lesions in the general population and are at slightly higher risk than a common nevus in predisposition to melanoma formation.[49] Most melanomas form in the absence of a benign nevus precursor and instead likely initiate from melanocytes or melanocyte stem cells and evolve first as intermediate lesions that histologically may be difficult to distinguish from a dysplastic nevus before progression to frank MIS or invasive melanoma.[50] Lentigo maligna melanoma (LMM) offers an example of this trajectory of melanoma with slow and prolonged expansion at the stage of MIS before rare progression to invasive melanoma. Nodular melanomas grow very rapidly and, in most cases, in the absence of an apparent precursor lesion.[51] It is thought that nodular melanoma is derived from a melanocyte or melanocyte stem cell that accumulates mutations that predispose to melanomagenesis and that is prone to melanoma formation after a second hit of an activating mutation in the mitogen-activated protein kinase (MAPK) pathway.[50]

Clinical and Histologic Classification of Melanoma

Four major variants of primary cutaneous melanoma have been classically described: superficial spreading melanoma, nodular melanoma, LMM, and acral lentiginous melanoma (**Fig. 3**). Different growth patterns characterize the clinical and pathologic features of early melanoma formation in these groups, but prognosis is similar for all 4 groups when normalized for depth of invasion (Breslow depth) at the time of diagnosis and treatment.[52] Although most melanomas are pigmented, about 5% to 10% of

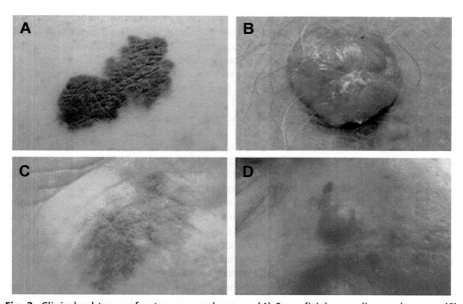

Fig. 3. Clinical subtypes of cutaneous melanoma. (*A*) Superficial spreading melanoma. (*B*) Nodular melanoma (*C*) LMM. (*D*) Amelanotic melanoma. (*From* Klebanov, N. et al. Clinical spectrum of cutaneous melanoma morphology. J Am Acad Dermatol 80(1), 178-188 (2019); with permission.)

cutaneous melanomas are amelanotic (see **Fig. 3**). Lack of pigmentation often delays diagnosis, thereby worsening prognosis, but when normalized for Breslow depth the prognosis of amelanotic lesions does not differ from pigmented melanoma.[53,54]

Superficial spreading melanoma (SSM) is the most common type of melanoma (60%–70% in fair-skinned populations). Clinically, SSMs show the hallmark ABCD melanoma features: asymmetry, irregular borders, color variegation, and increased diameter.[55] Typically, SSM has a prolonged (months to years) radial growth phase characterized by intraepidermal expansion without dermal invasion that proceeds to a vertical growth phase that is associated with dermal invasion and poorer prognosis. Nodular melanoma is most commonly located on chronically sun-exposed areas such as the head and neck. On histology, nodular melanomas show a vertical growth phase only and are thought to occur in the absence of a radial growth phase. They grow rapidly and usually present at an advanced Breslow depth. For this reason, nodular melanomas represent only 15% to 20% of primary melanomas but are responsible for more than 40% of melanoma deaths.[56,57] LMM occurs primarily in elderly patients on chronically sun-damaged (CSD) skin of the face. LMM is derived from an in situ lentigo maligna (LM) precursor that presents as a slowly enlarging and changing brown to black macule with irregular borders. About 5% of in situ LMs progress to LMM.[58]

A more recently proposed classification of cutaneous melanoma is based on whether it originated from CSD skin (CSD melanoma) or not (non-CSD melanoma).[59–61] CSD melanoma arises predominately in patients more than 55 years of age on areas of the head, neck, and dorsal extremities that are clinically photodamaged and histologically show evidence of solar elastosis and are enriched for nodular melanoma and LMM subtypes.[61,62] Non-CSD melanomas usually originate from areas of skin that are intermittently exposed to sun, such as the trunk and proximal extremities of younger individuals (<55 years of age), and in individuals with numerous nevi that do not show marked solar elastosis. Non-CSD melanomas are enriched for SSM subtypes and for melanomas arising from a benign nevus precursor.[61,63,64] Overall, this model suggests that non-CSD melanomas are initiated by intense intermittent sun exposure in patients whose melanocytes have more proliferative potential, whereas CSD melanomas are initiated mainly by exogenous stimulus of chronic UV exposure.[60] CSD melanomas show a higher mutational burden and are less likely to be associated with BRAF^{V600E} mutations (instead showing non-V600E BRAF mutations or mutations in neurofibromin 1 [NF1], NRAS, or KIT), whereas non-CSD melanomas are associated with a more moderate mutational burden and increased frequency of BRAF^{V600E} mutations.[65–69]

Acral lentiginous melanoma (ALM) occurs on the palms, soles, and within the nail apparatus. ALM incidence is similar among racial groups, but ALM is the predominant melanoma subtype in people with darker skin types, because SSM, nodular melanoma, and LMM are rare in nonwhite populations.[70] ALM presents clinically with gradual changes in size, shape, and color, similarly to SSM and LMM. Although a subset of nail-associated melanomas have been associated with a UV signature, most acral melanomas have a lower mutational burden, absent UV signature, and a higher number of genomic aberrations than nonacral melanomas.[67,71] There is some evidence that ALMs occur in areas of prior trauma and are more common in areas of chronic mechanical stress (eg, high-pressure areas of the plantar foot)[72]

There are several rare variants of cutaneous melanoma. Spitzoid melanomas show histologic features suggestive of benign Spitz nevi and are at times difficult to distinguish from their benign counterparts based on histology and molecular genetics.[73,74] Desmoplastic melanomas (DMs) occur on chronically sun-exposed skin and show extremely high mutational burdens.[75] Clinically, DMs manifest heterogeneously, often as flesh-colored, amelanotic, low-MITF–expressing nodules.[76] DMs are less aggressive than conventional melanomas and also have high response rates to anti–programmed cell death protein 1 (PD-1) immunotherapy, perhaps because of the large mutation/neoantigen burden.[77]

Melanoma can also occur on noncutaneous sites. Uveal melanomas are derived from melanocytes in the uvea (pigmented tissues of the eye below the sclera and cornea, comprising iris, choroid, and ciliary body).[78] Mucosal melanomas occur near the mucocutaneous junction of the oral cavity, pharynx, vagina, and anus. They account for approximately 1% of melanomas and are often diagnosed at advanced stages. Response of uveal and mucosal melanomas to immunotherapy has not been well studied, because these rare tumors are often excluded from clinical trial protocols, but they may respond less well because of lower UV-mutational burdens.[79] Melanoma of unknown primary (MUP) presents as a distant metastasis without a known primary lesion.[80] Recent studies have shown that MUPs have a high mutational burden with strong UV signature, validating the prevailing hypothesis that MUPs arise from regressed or unrecognized primary cutaneous melanoma.[81]

Clinical and Genetic Risk Factors for Melanoma

Major clinical risk factors for melanoma formation have been identified and include fair skin, increased number of melanocytic nevi, presence of dysplastic nevi, and a family history of melanoma. Twin studies have suggested that genetic susceptibility plays a large role in melanoma risk and about 5% to 10% of melanomas occur in patients with a known family history.[82] Germline mutations have been identified that account for a subset of familial melanomas. CDKN2A mutations are most common and occur in about 30% of melanoma families with 3 or more cases.[83–85] Germline mutations in CDK4, MITF, and genes regulating telomere maintenance (TERT, TERF21P, POT1, ACD) have been identified, but each explain less than 1% of familial melanoma cases.[22,83,86–89]

Numerous genome-wide association studies have identified genes that correlate with clinical risk factors that confer melanoma risk in the general population.[90–94] Although these gene loci individually have modest effects on melanoma risk, there is evidence that combinatorial assessment may allow risk stratification.[95] Moreover, identification of these risk genes gives insight into the biological processes that regulate melanoma development. Polymorphisms in genes associated with fair skin pigmentation also confer melanoma risk, including MC1R, ASIP, SLC45A2, and TYR.[91] Interestingly, many of the pigment-related melanoma risk loci also confer risk for cutaneous squamous cell carcinoma (SCC) formation, reaffirming a common link of UV exposure in melanoma and SCC.[93] Other melanoma risk genes are also associated with risk of an increased number of nevi and include MTAP-CDKN2A, PLA2G6, TERT, and IRF4, suggesting that biological processes leading to nevus formation also predispose to melanoma formation.[94]

UV exposure has long been identified as a strong melanoma risk factor. Epidemiologic studies have strongly implicated intermittent UV exposure and severe sunburns during childhood and early adulthood as strong risk factors.[96,97] Indoor artificial tanning devices that deliver primarily high-dose UVA spectrum (320–400 nM) radiation are also linked dose dependently to melanoma risk.[98] Direct photochemical interaction of UVB spectrum (280–320 nM) radiation with DNA leads to formation of stereotypical nucleotide adducts termed cyclobutane pyrimidine dimers, which, when repaired, incorrectly lead to transition of cytosine to thymidine at a dipyrimidine site (ie, UV signature mutations).[99] Recent exome sequencing studies have shown that, similar to other forms of skin cancer, cutaneous nonacral melanomas are characterized by a preponderance of UV signature mutations[71] (**Fig. 4**).

UV also drives other processes that contribute to melanoma formation. For example, the nucleotide changes responsible for BRAF^{V600E} and several common NRAS mutations do not display a UV signature, and may be caused by either UV-dependent or UV-independent mechanisms.[100] UVA spectrum radiation drives reactive oxygen production, which can lead to oxidative damage to DNA, lipids, and proteins.[101] Data from animal models show that UV induces inflammatory responses involving macrophages and neutrophils that can promote melanocyte cell survival, immunoevasion, and angiotropism.[102–104]

Melanoma Invasion, Lymph Node Spread, and Metastasis

As described earlier, most variants of melanoma show a radial growth phase with minimal invasion, followed by a vertical growth phase with dermal invasion. For all subtypes of primary melanoma, the risk of metastasis and death is most closely correlated with depth of invasion (Breslow depth) at the time of diagnosis and treatment. Because most melanomas are localized at the time of diagnosis (stage I and stage II), these common lesions that individually carry low risk lead to a large burden of melanoma fatalities. Many studies have examined indicators other than Breslow depth that might identify local melanomas at higher risk of metastasis, although the eighth edition AJCC (American Joint Committee on Cancer) guidelines list only tumor ulceration as an independent risk factor. Mitotic index was removed from these most

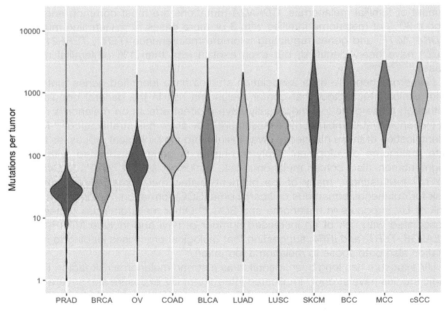

Fig. 4. Mutational burden in cancer is highest in cutaneous melanoma and UV-induced non-melanoma skin cancers. Mutation per tumor data from exome sequencing for prostate (PRAD), breast (BRCA), ovarian (OV), colorectal (COAD), bladder (BLCA), lung adenocarcinoma (LUAD), lung squamous cell (LUSC), and melanoma (SKCM) basal cell carcinoma (BCC), cutaneous SCC (cSCC), and polyomavirus-negative Merkel cell carcinoma (MCC). (*Data from* Refs.[240–244])

recent AJCC guidelines, because evidence does not support it as an independent risk factor for melanoma-specific survival. Microscopic lymphatic invasion and angiotropism have been shown to be associated with adverse clinical outcome but are not widely used in the clinical setting.[105] Several studies have identified specific gene expression signatures suggested to be associated with clinical risk in early melanomas.[106–111] Microenvironmental interactions are likely involved in melanoma invasion and metastasis, but, overall, this area of research remains underexplored. RXRα loss in keratinocytes strongly activates melanoma formation in mouse models and, similarly, loss of the hemidesmosomal protein desmoglein in keratinocytes increases MITF-driven pigmentation and melanomalike changes within melanocytes.[112–115]

Melanoma Metastasis

In contrast with nonmelanoma skin cancers such as basal cell carcinoma and SCCs, melanoma shows a high predilection for local, regional, and distant metastasis. As discussed earlier, the risk of metastasis correlates with depth of invasion and ulceration of the primary lesion. The early steps of metastasis in cancer have been well delineated and represent a series of steps of invasion, angiogenesis, extravasation, dissemination, and colonization of target organs.

Metastasis is often thought of as a linear process from local disease to nodal metastasis to distant metastasis. However, similar to other forms of cancer, several observations suggest that distant metastasis may occur in parallel with local disease progression in melanoma. First, patients with node-negative disease or who undergo sentinel lymph node basin resection can present with distant metastatic disease, and complete lymph node dissection has not been shown to offer survival benefit in node-positive patients.[116] Circulating tumor cells are also found in patients who present with local or regional disease.[117] Numerous reports describe the transfer of melanoma from organ transplant to recipient, even when the transplant was performed many years after the donor was diagnosed with thin melanoma.[118,119] This finding suggests that early distant metastatic seeding may be a common event, and clinically detectable distant metastasis is likely kept under control through a combination of microenvironmental and immune factors.

Overall, the search for metastasis-specific genetic perturbations in melanoma has been unfruitful, although copy number alterations, MITF amplification, TERT promoter mutation, and CDKN2A loss occur at higher frequencies in metastatic melanomas compared with primary melanomas.[120] Similarly although BAP1 mutation is associated with metastatic risk of uveal melanoma, this occurs early in primary disease progression and is not a specific feature of metastasis.[121,122] Several proteins, including NEDD9, have been suggested to play important roles in melanoma metastasis.[123] Melanoma has a predilection for central nervous system (CNS)/brain metastasis, resulting in high morbidity and resistance to therapy.[124–126] A recent study showed that immunosuppression and oxidative phosphorylation–related gene signatures were enriched in human melanoma CNS metastases, providing possible new therapeutic targets.[127]

MOLECULAR SIGNALING IN MELANOMA
Mitogen-Activated Protein Kinase Signaling

The MAPK signaling pathway is of central importance to the pathogenesis of many forms of cancer, in particular lung adenocarcinoma, colorectal adenocarcinoma, and melanoma. Canonical MAPK signaling occurs downstream of growth factor ligand binding to a receptor tyrosine kinase. This binding leads to recruitment of signaling adapters, including GRB2 and SHC, resulting in recruitment of RAS and conversion of inactive GDP-bound RAS (RAS-GDP) to active GTP-bound RAS (RAS-GTP) (see **Fig. 2**). RAS-GTP can activate several downstream signaling pathways, including the RAF–MAPK kinase (MEK)–MAPK cascade. Briefly, RAS binds to the RAS-binding domain of RAF, triggering RAF dimerization and activation. Phosphorylation of MEK by RAF leads to its activation and subsequent activating phosphorylation of MAPK. Activation of MAPK, also known as extracellular signal-regulated kinase (ERK), leads to phosphorylation of several substrates that promote cell cycle progression and cell survival in melanoma and other cancers.

MAPK activation in melanoma cells also results in the inhibition of apoptosis. This process has been shown to occur most commonly through regulation of proapoptotic and antiapoptotic BCL2 family member proteins, and, in particular, downregulation of the proapoptotic factor BIM.[128,129] It has recently been shown that BRAF inhibitors (BRAFi) paradoxically decrease the levels of the antiapoptotic factor NOXA, leading to targetable dependence on the proapoptotic factor MCL-1.[130]

BRAF

Recurrent activating mutations in BRAF are present in more than 50% of cutaneous melanomas.[71,131] These mutations most commonly (90%) lead to substitution for valine at codon 600 with glutamic acid (V600E). Less common mutations include other substitutions at codon 600 (eg, V600K), as well as other rare recurrent mutations that activate BRAF function (eg, G469R). Oncogenic BRAF mutation leads to constitutive BRAF activity and downstream activation of MEK and MAPK without the need for RAS/RAF engagement.[132,133] BRAF[V600E] mutations occur more commonly in nevus-associated melanoma, truncal location, and younger patients, whereas BRAF[V600K] mutations are more commonly linked to chronic UV exposure in chronically sun-exposed areas of the head and neck.[134,135] Genomic BRAF fusions leading to constitutive activation occur in 3% to 5% of melanomas, particularly in pan-negative (NRAS, BRAF, and NF1 negative) tumors.[136–138] Both BRAF[V600E] and BRAF[V600K] have been shown to be inhibited by mutation-specific small molecule BRAF inhibitors (BRAFi). Two such agents, vemurafenib and dabrafenib, have achieved US Food and Drug Administration (FDA) approval as single-use agents and in combination with MEK inhibitors (MEKi) for treatment of BRAF mutant melanoma, whereas a third agent, binimetinib, has been FDA approved for combination therapy with MEKi.[139–141] MEKi monotherapy has limited efficacy in BRAF[V600E]-mutated melanoma, but may offer some benefit in tumors with non-V600E BRAF mutations or BRAF fusions.[142]

NRAS/NF1

Recurrent activating mutation of NRAS is common in melanoma (15%–20%), with most mutations occurring at codon 61 (Q61R, Q61K, Q61L) and a small fraction occurring at codon 12. NRAS mutation activates the MAPK signaling cascade; however, although NRAS mutant melanoma cell lines are sensitive to MEK inhibition, single-agent MEK inhibitors in clinical trials offer only modest clinical benefit, fueling interest in combination therapies.[143,144] Because NRAS also activates the phosphoinositol-3-kinase (PI3K)–AKT pathway, combination therapy with PI3K inhibition showed promising in vitro efficacy to forestall MEKi resistance, but toxicities associated with this combination have prevented translation to clinical use.[145] CDK4 was identified as a mediator of MEKi resistance in NRAS mutant melanoma, although, clinically, dual MEK and CDK4/6 inhibition is also limited by side effects that require reduced dosing, resulting in decreased efficacy and susceptibility to development of resistance.[146,147]

A recent article identifies the serine/threonine kinase STK19 as an upstream NRAS regulator that may offer a novel therapeutic target.[148]

The tumor suppressor gene NF1 promotes conversion of active RAS-GTP to inactive RAS-GDP. Loss-of-function NF1 mutations occur in 10% to 15% of melanomas and lead to MAPK and PI3K activation.[71,149,150] Evidence suggests that NF1 mutant melanomas may be responsive to similar treatments as NRAS mutant melanoma.[151] About one-third of melanomas lack driver mutations in BRAF, NRAS, or NF1 (pan-negative or triple negative).

PTEN/Phosphoinositol-3-Kinase Signaling Pathway

PI3Ks represent 3 classes of multisubunit kinases that generate specific phosphoinositides. Only class I PI3K phosphorylates phosphatidylinositol (4,5)-bisphosphate (PIP2) to phosphatidylinositol (3,4,5)-trisphosphate (PIP3), a key second messenger that leads to downstream activation of the serine/threonine kinase Akt. Activated Akt promotes several cellular pathways involved in cell proliferation, survival, and angiogenesis. One of the key pathways regulated by Akt activation is the mammalian target of rapamycin (mTOR) complexes 1 and 2 (mTORC1 and mTORC2) through inhibition of the negative regulator tuberous sclerosis complex (TSC1/TSC2). Activation of mTORC1 and mTORC2 then leads to several cellular events and has been shown to overcome BRAF^{V600E}-induced growth arrest.[152] mTORC1 activation leads to phosphorylation of the ribosomal protein S6 (phospho-S6), a hallmark of mTOR activation that promotes cell growth and survival and has been identified as a node for resistance to targeted therapy.[153,154]

In melanoma, PI3K can be activated by NRAS mutation, mutation of NF1, or loss of the tumor suppressor PTEN. PTEN acts as a lipid phosphatase to convert PIP3 to PIP2 to antagonize PI3K function.[155] PTEN loss by deletion, mutation, or epigenetic dysregulation potentiates PI3K, occurs in up to 30% of melanomas, and is most commonly associated with BRAF^{V600E} mutation, underscoring the strong roles of both MAPK and PI3K activation for melanomagenesis.[156–158] PTEN also can act independently of PI3K and AKT, and there is some evidence that AKT-independent effects of PTEN are important in melanomagenesis.[159]

RAC1

The RAC1 GTPase plays key roles in regulating the cytoskeleton and numerous other cellular pathways, including MAPK and PI3K signaling.[160] Recurrent activating RAC1 mutations have been identified in approximately 5% of melanoma by exome sequencing.[161,162] Interestingly, mutation in PREX2, a GEF that negatively regulates RAC1, is common in melanoma.[163] RAC1 activation and/or PREX2 loss leads to direct activation of PI3K, promotes melanoma in mouse models, and contributes to therapy resistence.[164–166]

CDKN2A

The CDKN2A locus encodes 2 proteins, p16(INK4A) and p14(ARF), both of which serve as tumor suppressors in melanoma and other cancers. p16(INK4A) binds CDK4 and CDK6 to block their ability to stimulate cell cycle progression, whereas p14(ARF) protects p53 from degradation. CDKN2A is silenced by deletion, mutation, and/or methylation in up to 90% of melanomas. CDKN2A and CDK4 somatic mutations contribute to familial melanoma. CDKN2A loss occurs during early stages of melanoma progression (development of MIS and invasive melanoma), and recent elegant studies showed that CDKN2A loss in primary human melanocytes leads to depression of a BRN2-mediated cell invasiveness program.[167] Interestingly, most CDKN2A deletions result in loss of neighboring loci such as CDKN2B and MTAP. CDKN2B encodes the CDK (cyclin-dependent kinase) inhibitor p15, and it has been shown that CDKN2B loss promotes melanomagenesis.[168] MTAP plays a key role in the methionine salvage pathway, and MTAP loss leads to therapeutic dependency on PRMT5 methyltransferase.[169,170]

Telomerase Reverse Transcriptase Promoter Mutations

TERT encodes the catalytic subunit of telomerase. Recurrent TERT promoter mutations were identified by whole-genome sequencing and are present in 50% of cutaneous nonacral melanomas, and at lower frequencies in acral and mucosal melanomas.[88,171,172] TERT promoter mutations in melanoma show UV signatures and act to create de novo consensus ETS transcription factor binding sites, leading to increased TERT promoter activity, telomerase expression, and promotion of replicative capacity of the cell. TERT promoter mutations are associated with high-risk primary melanoma features (ulceration, advanced Breslow depth, rapid primary tumor growth), are independently associated with poor prognosis and risk of metastasis, and also contribute to familial and sporadic melanoma risk.[88,171,173–175] It has since been recognized that functionally similar TERT promoter mutations occur in other forms of cancer.[176]

Molecular Alteration and Signaling Specific to Acral Lentiginous, Mucosal, and Chronically Sun-Damaged Melanoma

MAPK pathway activating mutations such as NRAS and BRAF occur in CSD and acral melanomas; however, the frequency is much lower in mucosal melanomas. In addition, BRAF mutations that do occur are predominately non-BRAF^{V600E} mutations.[177] Inactivating NF1 mutations and concurrent mutations in other genes related to Ras activation, such as RASA2, occur frequently in BRAF/NRAS wild-type cutaneous melanomas, and activate the MAPK pathway.[149]

KIT

KIT (c-Kit) is a receptor tyrosine kinase that binds KIT ligand (KITLG) (also known as steel factor or stem cell factor [SCF]) to mediate important roles during melanocyte development. Recurrent mutations and genomic amplifications of KIT that result in constitutive activation of the receptor are associated with several forms of cancer, including acral lentiginous, mucosal, and CSD melanomas, occurring in up to 30% to 40% of these cases.[178] KIT activates numerous signaling pathways, including the MAPK pathway, and has been shown to lead to MITF functional upregulation.[179]

Molecular Alteration and Signaling Specific to Uveal Melanoma

Recurrent activating mutations of the G protein alpha subunit (GNA) family members GNAQ and GNA11 occur in a mutually exclusive fashion and act as key driver mutations in almost all uveal nevi and uveal melanomas.[180,181] The driver mutations lead to a constitutively activating conformation of the Gα subunit (encoded by these genes) of Gq heterotrimeric G proteins. Hotspot mutations occur less commonly in CYSLTR2 to activate endogenous Gαq.[182] Activation of Gq proteins contributes to melanomagenesis by activation of protein kinase C (PKC) and subsequent activation of MAPK and YAP1 pathways.[78] Rare activating mutations of the PKC regulator PLBC4 are mutually exclusive to GNAQ/GNA11/CYSLTR2 mutations, reinforcing the importance of the PKC pathway in uveal melanoma.[183] Inactivating and truncating mutations of BAP1 are detected in up to 40% of uveal melanomas and are highly associated with metastatic risk, whereas mutations of EIFAX and SF3B1 are mutually exclusive to BAP1 mutation and are associated with low-risk subtypes.[184]

Epigenetic Perturbations in Melanomas

Epigenetic modifications represent somatically inherited modifications of chromatin components (including both DNA and histone proteins) that alter gene transcription without changing nucleotide sequences. Disruption of the epigenetic landscape is common in melanoma. Aberrant DNA methylation was identified as a hallmark of melanoma, and many studies have suggested it plays a major role in melanoma progression.[185]

Chromatin states that are permissive or repressive for gene transcription are regulated by posttranslational modification of histone proteins by acetylation, methylation, phosphorylation, and/or ubiquitination. SETDB1 acts to promote repressive trimethylation of H3K9 residues. Genomic amplification of SETDB1 promotes melanomagenesis and offered one of the first examples of the important roles of chromatin factors in oncogenesis.[186] The histone methyltransferase G9a catalyzes repressive H3K9 dimethylation. Rare recurrent mutations and more common genomic amplification of G9a (*EHMT2*) promote melanomagenesis through regulation of DKK1, a repressor of WNT signaling.[187] The polycomb 2 (PRC2) complex catalyzes H3K27 trimethylation, a histone modification associated with transcriptional repression. The catalytic PRC2 subunit EZH2 is recurrently mutated or amplified in a subset of melanomas and has been validated to drive melanoma in a mouse model.[169]

SWI/SNF comprises a subfamily of large, heterogeneous, multisubunit complexes (BAF and PBAF) that reposition nucleosome complexes to allow access for gene transcription (chromatin remodeling). SWI/SNF complexes play critical roles in regulation of gene transcription, in particular at enhancer and superenhancer sites, and have been shown to also directly modulate the activity of epigenetic regulators.[188] SWI/SNF complexes also play important roles in the DNA damage response and maintenance of genome integrity.[189,190] SWI/SNF component genes are among the most highly mutated in cancers, including melanoma.[162] The exact mechanism by which mutation of SWI/SNF complex components contributes to cancer formation is unclear, although it has been shown that SWI/SNF mutations may confer unique vulnerabilities and therapy targets.[191]

BIOLOGY OF THERAPY RESISTANCE IN MELANOMA
Biology of Targeted Therapy Resistance

Targeted therapy with BRAFi leads to a dramatic response rate and offers survival benefit in most cases, but patients almost uniformly relapse and eventually succumb to disease.[192] Several mechanisms of resistance have been identified and can be broadly characterized as (1) MAPK reactivation, (2) upregulation of survival pathways, and (3) development of dedifferentiated/MITF^{low} cell state.

Genomic and genetic alterations leading to MAPK reactivation are noted in up to 60% of melanomas that develop resistance to BRAFi.[193–195] These alterations include mutation of NRAS; amplification, fusion, or alternative splice mutation of BRAF; mutation of MEK1 or MEK2; and NF1 loss.[196–199] Genetic alterations leading to upregulation of the PI3K-PTEN-AKT pathway also occur in a lower percentage of cases.[198] Combination therapy with MEKi was designed to decrease the chance of developing MAPK reactivation–induced resistance.[46] Although combination therapy offers survival benefits, relapse is still nearly universal and similar genetic resistance mechanisms have been identified.[200–202]

Several survival pathways have been shown to be involved in targeted therapy resistance. p21-activated kinase (PAK) upregulation was shown to mediate resistance to BRAFi/MEKi therapy through β-catenin phosphorylation and mTOR pathway activation.[203] Several studies have shown upregulation of growth factor receptors (EGFR, PDGFR, EPHA2, AXL, NGF) in the setting of BRAFi resistance; however, some evidence suggests that these may act largely as markers of the MITF[low]/therapy-resistant state (discussed later). The best-validated survival pathway in targeted therapy resistance is upregulation of MITF expression and subsequent activation of lineage-specific survival pathways. This mechanism was first identified in overexpression screening of melanoma cell lines.[204] It has since been validated that a subset (20%–40%) of BRAFi-resistant tumors show MITF upregulation.[205–207] It has been suggested that, in the setting of BRAFi, MITF upregulation may occur through transcriptional control of the MITF regulator PAX3.[205]

In contrast with MITF upregulation, it has become increasingly clear that phenotypic plasticity leading to predominance of a MITF[low] state is a key driver of targeted therapy resistance in many tumors. Melanoma cell lines were initially found to possess either a proliferative (MITF[high]) or an invasive (MITF[low]) expression signature, and, in tumors, switching from an MITF[high] to an MITF[low] state may accompany metastatic progression of melanoma.[208,209]

MITF[low] melanoma cell lines express high levels of the tyrosinase kinase receptor AXL, and MITF[low]/AXL[high] cell lines are intrinsically resistant to BRAF and MEK inhibition.[210–213] The MITF[low]/AXL[high] phenotype has been characterized in bulk transcriptomic sequencing in human melanomas, and such tumors are intrinsically resistant to BRAF inhibitor.[71] Interestingly, single cell RNA sequencing of human melanomas showed that tumors identified as MITF[high] from bulk sequencing contained cells showing gradients of expression that include low-MITF cells.[206,214] Although there is some evidence that resistance can develop through selective growth advantage of preexisting MITF[low] cells, it seems that, in most cases, drug treatment results in phenotypic transition from an MITF[high] to an MITF[low] state.[215–218] MITF[high] and MITF[low] melanomas are associated with distinct epigenetic signatures, but mechanisms underlying switching or maintenance of these epigenetic states are unclear.[210] It has been shown that the inflammation and stromal signaling in the tumor microenvironment can contribute to dedifferentiation and therapy resistance.[219–223] The MITF[low]/dedifferentiated state shows unique therapy sensitivities that may allow prevention of therapy resistance.[151,207,217,218,224] It is anticipated that a better understanding of this epigenetic state may identify unique vulnerabilities that enable enhanced therapies.

Biology of Immunotherapy Response and Immunotherapy Resistance

The advent of immunotherapy has transformed treatment of many cancers, perhaps most strikingly melanoma. Treatment with α-PD-1 and alpha-cytotoxic T lymphocyte–associated protein 4 (α-CTLA-4) leads to durable responses in up to 40% of patients, after the previous best treatments for melanoma provided ~5% long-term survival. Immunotherapy has also shown benefit in an adjuvant setting for stage III melanoma.[225] However, many patients still show no initial response to therapy (innate resistance), whereas approximately 40% with a good response ultimately relapse (acquired resistance).[226]

Several mechanisms have been shown to lead to immunotherapy resistance in melanoma. These mechanisms include loss of antigen presentation machinery and deficiency in interferon signaling.[227–229] Interestingly, there is substantial evidence that the MITF[low]/dedifferentiated phenotype also leads to therapy resistance.[192,230–233] Single-cell analyses from patients with melanoma have shown transcriptional signatures in both immune cells and tumor cells that correspond with response to therapy.[234,235] Studies from animal models have suggested that perturbations of epigenetic pathways can dramatically alter response to immunotherapy, and further research efforts may allow targeting of epigenetic pathways for therapeutic benefit.[236–239]

SUMMARY

In the last decade, there has been a revolution in understanding the molecular complexity of melanoma biology as well as major advances in therapy that benefit survival of patients with melanoma. However, resistance to therapy remains a major hurdle in melanoma care. Better understanding of mechanisms of residence to therapy, including the MITF^{low}/dedifferentiated resistance phenotype, may provide better therapeutic opportunities in melanoma.

ACKNOWLEDGMENTS

The authors grateful acknowledge Dr C. Thomas Powell for expert assistance with article preparation. They also acknowledge support to the Fisher Laboratory from NIH grants 2P01 CA163222-06, 5R01CA222871-02, 5R01AR072304-03, and 5R01 AR043369-23, and funding from the Dr. Miriam and Sheldon G. Adelson Medical Research Foundation.

DISCLOSURE

Dr D.E. Fisher has a financial interest in Soltego, Inc, a company developing SIK inhibitors for topical skin darkening treatments that might be used for a broad set of human applications. Dr D.E. Fisher's interests were reviewed and are managed by Massachusetts General Hospital and Partners Healthcare in accordance with their conflict of interest policies.

REFERENCES

1. Moyer FH. Genetic variations in the fine structure and ontogeny of mouse melanin granules. Am Zool 1966;6(1):43–66.
2. Wu X, Hammer JA. Melanosome transfer: it is best to give and receive. Curr Opin Cell Biol 2014;29:1–7.
3. Wu X, Bowers B, Rao K, et al. Visualization of melanosome dynamics within wild-type and dilute melanocytes suggests a paradigm for myosin V function In vivo. J Cell Biol 1998;143(7):1899–918.
4. Gates RR, Zimmermann AA. Comparison of skin color with melanin content. J Invest Dermatol 1953;21(6):339–48.
5. Sturm RA. Molecular genetics of human pigmentation diversity. Hum Mol Genet 2009;18(R1):R9–17.
6. Prota G. Recent advances in the chemistry of melanogenesis in mammals. J Invest Dermatol 1980;75(1):122–7.
7. Robbins LS, Nadeau JH, Johnson KR, et al. Pigmentation phenotypes of variant extension locus alleles result from point mutations that alter MSH receptor function. Cell 1993;72(6):827–34.
8. Cui R, Widlund HR, Feige E, et al. Central role of p53 in the suntan response and pathologic hyperpigmentation. Cell 2007;128(5):853–64.
9. Millington GW. Proopiomelanocortin (POMC): the cutaneous roles of its melanocortin products and receptors. Clin Exp Dermatol 2006;31(3):407–12.

10. Mujahid N, Liang Y, Murakami R, et al. A UV-Independent Topical Small-Molecule Approach for Melanin Production in Human Skin. Cell Rep 2017; 19(11):2177–84.

11. Horike N, Kumagai A, Shimono Y, et al. Downregulation of SIK2 expression promotes the melanogenic program in mice. Pigment Cell Melanoma Res 2010; 23(6):809–19.

12. Miller AJ, Du J, Rowan S, et al. Transcriptional regulation of the melanoma prognostic marker melastatin (TRPM1) by MITF in melanocytes and melanoma. Cancer Res 2004;64(2):509–16.

13. Du J, Miller AJ, Widlund HR, et al. MLANA/MART1 and SILV/PMEL17/GP100 are transcriptionally regulated by MITF in melanocytes and melanoma. Am J Pathol 2003;163(1):333–43.

14. Haq R, Yokoyama S, Hawryluk EB, et al. BCL2A1 is a lineage-specific antiapoptotic melanoma oncogene that confers resistance to BRAF inhibition. Proc Natl Acad Sci U S A 2013;110(11):4321–6.

15. McGill GG, Horstmann M, Widlund HR, et al. Bcl2 regulation by the melanocyte master regulator Mitf modulates lineage survival and melanoma cell viability. Cell 2002;109(6):707–18.

16. Du J, Widlund HR, Horstmann MA, et al. Critical role of CDK2 for melanoma growth linked to its melanocyte-specific transcriptional regulation by MITF. Cancer Cell 2004;6(6):565–76.

17. Hodgkinson CA, Moore KJ, Nakayama A, et al. Mutations at the mouse microphthalmia locus are associated with defects in a gene encoding a novel basic-helix-loop-helix-zipper protein. Cell 1993;74(2):395–404.

18. Hughes AE, Newton VE, Liu XZ, et al. A gene for Waardenburg syndrome type 2 maps close to the human homologue of the microphthalmia gene at chromosome 3p12-p14.1. Nat Genet 1994;7(4):509–12.

19. Tsherniak A, Vazquez F, Montgomery PG, et al. Defining a cancer dependency map. Cell 2017;170(3):564–76.e16.

20. Davis IJ, Kim JJ, Ozsolak F, et al. Oncogenic MITF dysregulation in clear cell sarcoma: defining the MiT family of human cancers. Cancer Cell 2006;9(6): 473–84.

21. Garraway LA, Widlund HR, Rubin MA, et al. Integrative genomic analyses identify MITF as a lineage survival oncogene amplified in malignant melanoma. Nature 2005;436(7047):117–22.

22. Yokoyama S, Woods SL, Boyle GM, et al. A novel recurrent mutation in MITF predisposes to familial and sporadic melanoma. Nature 2011;480(7375):99–103.

23. Bertolotto C, Lesueur F, Giuliano S, et al. A SUMOylation-defective MITF germline mutation predisposes to melanoma and renal carcinoma. Nature 2011; 480(7375):94–8.

24. Valverde P, Healy E, Jackson I, et al. Variants of the melanocyte-stimulating hormone receptor gene are associated with red hair and fair skin in humans. Nat Genet 1995;11(3):328–30.

25. Abdel-Malek Z, Scott MC, Suzuki I, et al. The melanocortin-1 receptor is a key regulator of human cutaneous pigmentation. Pigment Cell Res 2000;13 Suppl 8(Suppl 8):156–62.

26. Robles-Espinoza CD, Roberts ND, Chen S, et al. Germline MC1R status influences somatic mutation burden in melanoma. Nat Commun 2016;7:12064.

27. Valverde P, Healy E, Sikkink S, et al. The Asp84Glu variant of the melanocortin 1 receptor (MC1R) is associated with melanoma. Hum Mol Genet 1996;5(10): 1663–6.

28. D'Orazio JA, Nobuhisa T, Cui R, et al. Topical drug rescue strategy and skin protection based on the role of Mc1r in UV-induced tanning. Nature 2006; 443(7109):340–4.
29. Nobuhisa JS, Duffy DL, Box NF, et al. Melanocortin-1 receptor polymorphisms and risk of melanoma: is the association explained solely by pigmentation phenotype? Am J Hum Genet 2000;66(1):176–86.
30. Wendt J, Rauscher S, Burgstaller-Muehlbacher S, et al. Human determinants and the role of melanocortin-1 receptor variants in melanoma risk independent of UV radiation exposure. JAMA Dermatol 2016;152(7):776–82.
31. Roider EM, Fisher DE. Red Hair, Light Skin, and UV-Independent Risk for Melanoma Development in Humans. JAMA Dermatol 2016;152(7):751–3.
32. Mitra D, Luo X, Morgan A, et al. An ultraviolet-radiation-independent pathway to melanoma carcinogenesis in the red hair/fair skin background. Nature 2012; 491(7424):449–53.
33. Napolitano A, Panzella L, Monfrecola G, et al. Pheomelanin-induced oxidative stress: bright and dark chemistry bridging red hair phenotype and melanoma. Pigment Cell Melanoma Res 2014;27(5):721–33.
34. Michaloglou C, Vredeveld LC, Soengas MS, et al. BRAFE600-associated senescence-like cell cycle arrest of human naevi. Nature 2005;436(7051): 720–4.
35. Jansen P, Cosgarea I, Murali R, et al. Frequent Occurrence of NRAS and BRAF Mutations in Human Acral Naevi. Cancers (Basel) 2019;11(4). https://doi.org/10.3390/cancers11040546.
36. Pollock PM, Harper UL, Hansen KS, et al. High frequency of BRAF mutations in nevi. Nat Genet 2003;33(1):19–20.
37. Krengel S, Scope A, Dusza SW, et al. New recommendations for the categorization of cutaneous features of congenital melanocytic nevi. J Am Acad Dermatol 2013;68(3):441–51.
38. Martins da Silva V, Martinez-Barrios E, Tell-Martí G, et al. Genetic abnormalities in large to giant congenital nevi: beyond NRAS mutations. J Invest Dermatol 2019;139(4):900–8.
39. Polubothu S, McGuire N, Al-Olabi L, et al. Does the gene matter? Genotype-phenotype and genotype-outcome associations in congenital melanocytic naevi. Br J Dermatol 2020;182(2):434–43.
40. Kinsler VA, O'Hare P, Bulstrode N, et al. Melanoma in congenital melanocytic naevi. Br J Dermatol 2017;176(5):1131–43.
41. Leikam C, Hufnagel A, Schartl M, et al. Oncogene activation in melanocytes links reactive oxygen to multinucleated phenotype and senescence. Oncogene 2008;27(56):7070–82.
42. Colebatch AJ, Ferguson P, Newell F, et al. Molecular genomic profiling of melanocytic nevi. J Invest Dermatol 2019;139(8):1762–8.
43. Stark MS, Tan JM, Tom L, et al. Whole-exome sequencing of acquired nevi identifies mechanisms for development and maintenance of benign neoplasms. J Invest Dermatol 2018;138(7):1636–44.
44. Melamed RD, Aydin IT, Rajan GS, et al. Genomic characterization of dysplastic nevi unveils implications for diagnosis of melanoma. J Invest Dermatol 2017; 137(4):905–9.
45. Tsao H, Bevona C, Goggins W, et al. The transformation rate of moles (melanocytic nevi) into cutaneous melanoma: a population-based estimate. Arch Dermatol 2003;139(3):282–8.

46. Shain AH, Joseph NM, Yu R, et al. Genomic and transcriptomic analysis reveals incremental disruption of key signaling pathways during melanoma evolution. Cancer Cell 2018;34(1):45–55.e4.

47. Shain AH, Yeh I, Kovalyshyn I, et al. The genetic evolution of melanoma from precursor lesions. N Engl J Med 2015;373(20):1926–36.

48. Bevona C, Goggins W, Quinn T, et al. Cutaneous melanomas associated with nevi. Arch Dermatol 2003;139(12):1620–4 [discussion: 1624].

49. Strazzula L, Vedak P, Hoang MP, et al. The utility of re-excising mildly and moderately dysplastic nevi: a retrospective analysis. J Am Acad Dermatol 2014;71(6):1071–6.

50. Shain AH, Bastian BC. From melanocytes to melanomas. Nat Rev Cancer 2016; 16(6):345–58.

51. Clark WH Jr, Ainsworth AM, Bernardino EA, et al. The developmental biology of primary human malignant melanomas. Semin Oncol 1975;2(2):83–103.

52. Breslow A. Thickness, cross-sectional areas and depth of invasion in the prognosis of cutaneous melanoma. Ann Surg 1970;172(5):902–8.

53. Moreau JF, Weissfeld JL, Ferris LK. Characteristics and survival of patients with invasive amelanotic melanoma in the USA. Melanoma Res 2013;23(5):408–13.

54. Thomas NE, Kricker A, Waxweiler WT, et al. Comparison of clinicopathologic features and survival of histopathologically amelanotic and pigmented melanomas: a population-based study. JAMA Dermatol 2014;150(12):1306–14.

55. Friedman RJ, Rigel DS, Kopf AW. Early detection of malignant melanoma: the role of physician examination and self-examination of the skin. CA Cancer J Clin 1985;35(3):130–51.

56. Shaikh WR, Xiong M, Weinstock MA. The contribution of nodular subtype to melanoma mortality in the United States, 1978 to 2007. Arch Dermatol 2012; 148(1):30–6.

57. Mar V, Roberts H, Wolfe R, et al. Nodular melanoma: a distinct clinical entity and the largest contributor to melanoma deaths in Victoria, Australia. J Am Acad Dermatol 2013;68(4):568–75.

58. Weinstock MA, Sober AJ. The risk of progression of lentigo maligna to lentigo maligna melanoma. Br J Dermatol 1987;116(3):303–10.

59. Whiteman DC, Pavan WJ, Bastian BC. The melanomas: a synthesis of epidemiological, clinical, histopathological, genetic, and biological aspects, supporting distinct subtypes, causal pathways, and cells of origin. Pigment Cell Melanoma Res 2011;24(5):879–97.

60. Whiteman DC, Parsons PG, Green AC. p53 expression and risk factors for cutaneous melanoma: a case-control study. Int J Cancer 1998;77(6):843–8.

61. Bastian BC. The molecular pathology of melanoma: an integrated taxonomy of melanocytic neoplasia. Annu Rev Pathol 2014;9:239–71.

62. Whiteman DC, Stickley M, Watt P, et al. Anatomic site, sun exposure, and risk of cutaneous melanoma. J Clin Oncol 2006;24(19):3172–7.

63. Newton-Bishop JA, Chang YM, Iles MM, et al. Melanocytic nevi, nevus genes, and melanoma risk in a large case-control study in the United Kingdom. Cancer Epidemiol Biomarkers Prev 2010;19(8):2043–54.

64. Olsen CM, Zens MS, Stukel TA, et al. Nevus density and melanoma risk in women: a pooled analysis to test the divergent pathway hypothesis. Int J Cancer 2009;124(4):937–44.

65. Hacker E, Olsen CM, Kvaskoff M, et al. Histologic and Phenotypic Factors and MC1R Status Associated with BRAF(V600E), BRAF(V600K), and NRAS

Mutations in a Community-Based Sample of 414 Cutaneous Melanomas. J Invest Dermatol 2016;136(4):829–37.

66. Mar VJ, Wong SQ, Li J, et al. BRAF/NRAS wild-type melanomas have a high mutation load correlating with histologic and molecular signatures of UV damage. Clin Cancer Res 2013;19(17):4589–98.

67. Curtin JA, Fridlyand J, Kageshita T, et al. Distinct sets of genetic alterations in melanoma. N Engl J Med 2005;353(20):2135–47.

68. Long GV, Menzies AM, Nagrial AM, et al. Prognostic and clinicopathologic associations of oncogenic BRAF in metastatic melanoma. J Clin Oncol 2011; 29(10):1239–46.

69. Sanna A, Harbst K, Johansson I, et al. Tumor genetic heterogeneity analysis of chronic sun-damaged melanoma. Pigment Cell Melanoma Res 2019;33(3):480.

70. Wang Y, Zhao Y, Ma S. Racial differences in six major subtypes of melanoma: descriptive epidemiology. BMC Cancer 2016;16:691.

71. Cancer Genome Atlas N. Genomic classification of cutaneous melanoma. Cell 2015;161(7):1681–96.

72. Basurto-Lozada P, Molina-Aguilar C, Castaneda-Garcia C, et al. Acral lentiginous melanoma: Basic facts, biological characteristics and research perspectives of an understudied disease. Pigment Cell Melanoma Res 2020. https://doi.org/10.1111/pcmr.12885.

73. Quan VL, Zhang B, Zhang Y, et al. Integrating next-generation sequencing with morphology improves prognostic and biologic classification of spitz neoplasms. J Invest Dermatol 2020;140(8):1599.

74. Wiesner T, He J, Yelensky R, et al. Kinase fusions are frequent in Spitz tumours and spitzoid melanomas. Nat Commun 2014;5:3116.

75. Shain AH, Garrido M, Botton T, et al. Exome sequencing of desmoplastic melanoma identifies recurrent NFKBIE promoter mutations and diverse activating mutations in the MAPK pathway. Nat Genet 2015;47(10):1194–9.

76. DeWane ME, Kelsey A, Oliviero M, et al. Melanoma on chronically sun-damaged skin: Lentigo maligna and desmoplastic melanoma. J Am Acad Dermatol 2019; 81(3):823–33.

77. Eroglu Z, Zaretsky JM, Hu-Lieskovan S, et al. High response rate to PD-1 blockade in desmoplastic melanomas. Nature 2018;553(7688):347–50.

78. Jager MJ, Shields CL, Cebulla CM, et al. Uveal melanoma. Nat Rev Dis Primers 2020;6(1):24.

79. Seth R, Messersmith H, Kaur V, et al. Systemic Therapy for Melanoma: ASCO Guideline. J Clin Oncol 2020. https://doi.org/10.1200/JCO.20.00198.

80. Song Y, Karakousis GC. Melanoma of unknown primary. J Surg Oncol 2019; 119(2):232–41.

81. Dutton-Regester K, Kakavand H, Aoude LG, et al. Melanomas of unknown primary have a mutation profile consistent with cutaneous sun-exposed melanoma. Pigment Cell Melanoma Res 2013;26(6):852–60.

82. Shekar SN, Duffy DL, Youl P, et al. A population-based study of Australian twins with melanoma suggests a strong genetic contribution to liability. J Invest Dermatol 2009;129(9):2211–9.

83. Zuo L, Weger J, Yang Q, et al. Germline mutations in the p16INK4a binding domain of CDK4 in familial melanoma. Nat Genet 1996;12(1):97–9.

84. FitzGerald MG, Harkin DP, Silva-Arrieta S, et al. Prevalence of germ-line mutations in p16, p19ARF, and CDK4 in familial melanoma: analysis of a clinic-based population. Proc Natl Acad Sci U S A 1996;93(16):8541–5.

85. Koh J, Enders GH, Dynlacht BD, et al. Tumour-derived p16 alleles encoding proteins defective in cell-cycle inhibition. Nature 1995;375(6531):506–10.
86. Shi J, Yang XR, Ballew B, et al. Rare missense variants in POT1 predispose to familial cutaneous malignant melanoma. Nat Genet 2014;46(5):482–6.
87. Robles-Espinoza CD, Harland M, Ramsay AJ, et al. POT1 loss-of-function variants predispose to familial melanoma. Nat Genet 2014;46(5):478–81.
88. Horn S, Figl A, Rachakonda PS, et al. TERT promoter mutations in familial and sporadic melanoma. Science 2013;339(6122):959–61.
89. Aoude LG, Pritchard AL, Robles-Espinoza CD, et al. Nonsense mutations in the shelterin complex genes ACD and TERF2IP in familial melanoma. J Natl Cancer Inst 2015;107(2). https://doi.org/10.1093/jnci/dju408.
90. Landi MT, Timothy Bishop D, MacGregor S, et al. Genome-wide association meta-analyses combining multiple risk phenotypes provide insights into the genetic architecture of cutaneous melanoma susceptibility. Nat Genet 2020. https://doi.org/10.1038/s41588-020-0611-8.
91. Law MH, Bishop DT, Lee JE, et al. Genome-wide meta-analysis identifies five new susceptibility loci for cutaneous malignant melanoma. Nat Genet 2015; 47(9):987–95.
92. Choi J, Xu M, Makowski MM, et al. A common intronic variant of PARP1 confers melanoma risk and mediates melanocyte growth via regulation of MITF. Nat Genet 2017;49(9):1326–35.
93. Sarin KY, Lin Y, Daneshjou R, et al. Genome-wide meta-analysis identifies eight new susceptibility loci for cutaneous squamous cell carcinoma. Nat Commun 2020;11(1):820.
94. Falchi M, Bataille V, Hayward NK, et al. Genome-wide association study identifies variants at 9p21 and 22q13 associated with development of cutaneous nevi. Nat Genet 2009;41(8):915–9.
95. Cho HG, Ransohoff KJ, Yang L, et al. Melanoma risk prediction using a multilocus genetic risk score in the Women's Health Initiative cohort. J Am Acad Dermatol 2018;79(1):36.e10.
96. Gandini S, Sera F, Cattaruzza MS, et al. Meta-analysis of risk factors for cutaneous melanoma: II. Sun exposure. Eur J Cancer 2005;41(1):45–60.
97. Whiteman DC, Whiteman CA, Green AC. Childhood sun exposure as a risk factor for melanoma: a systematic review of epidemiologic studies. Cancer Causes Control 2001;12(1):69–82.
98. Boniol M, Autier P, Boyle P, et al. Cutaneous melanoma attributable to sunbed use: systematic review and meta-analysis. BMJ 2012;345:e4757.
99. Brash DE. UV signature mutations. Photochem Photobiol 2015;91(1):15–26.
100. Thomas NE, Berwick M, Cordeiro-Stone M. Could BRAF mutations in melanocytic lesions arise from DNA damage induced by ultraviolet radiation? J Invest Dermatol 2006;126(8):1693–6.
101. de Gruijl FR. Photocarcinogenesis: Photocarcinogenesis: UVA vs UVB. Meth Enzymol 2000;319:359–66.
102. Viros A, Sanchez-Laorden B, Pedersen M, et al. Ultraviolet radiation accelerates BRAF-driven melanomagenesis by targeting TP53. Nature 2014;511(7510): 478–82.
103. Zaidi MR, Davis S, Noonan FP, et al. Interferon-γ links ultraviolet radiation to melanomagenesis in mice. Nature 2011;469(7331):548–53.
104. Handoko HY, Rodero MP, Boyle GM, et al. UVB-induced melanocyte proliferation in neonatal mice driven by CCR2-independent recruitment of Ly6c(low) MHCII(hi) macrophages. J Invest Dermatol 2013;133(7):1803–12.

105. Xu X, Gimotty PA, Guerry D, et al. Lymphatic invasion as a prognostic biomarker in primary cutaneous melanoma. Methods Mol Biol 2014;1102:275–86.
106. Gerami P, Cook RW, Wilkinson J, et al. Development of a prognostic genetic signature to predict the metastatic risk associated with cutaneous melanoma. Clin Cancer Res 2015;21(1):175–83.
107. Badal B, Solovyov A, Di Cecilia S, et al. Transcriptional dissection of melanoma identifies a high-risk subtype underlying TP53 family genes and epigenome deregulation. JCI Insight 2017;2(9). https://doi.org/10.1172/jci.insight.92102.
108. Kunz M, Löffler-Wirth H, Dannemann M, et al. RNA-seq analysis identifies different transcriptomic types and developmental trajectories of primary melanomas. Oncogene 2018;37(47):6136–51.
109. Nsengimana J, Laye J, Filia A, et al. Independent replication of a melanoma subtype gene signature and evaluation of its prognostic value and biological correlates in a population cohort. Oncotarget 2015;6(13):11683–93.
110. Thakur R, Laye JP, Lauss M, et al. Transcriptomic Analysis Reveals Prognostic Molecular Signatures of Stage I Melanoma. Clin Cancer Res 2019;25(24):7424–35.
111. Greenhaw BN, Covington KR, Kurley SJ, et al. Molecular risk prediction in cutaneous melanoma: a meta-analysis of the 31-gene expression profile prognostic test in 1,479 patients. J Am Acad Dermatol 2020;83(3):745.
112. Hyter S, Bajaj G, Liang X, et al. Loss of nuclear receptor RXRα in epidermal keratinocytes promotes the formation of Cdk4-activated invasive melanomas. Pigment Cell Melanoma Res 2010;23(5):635–48.
113. Chagani S, Wang R, Carpenter EL, et al. Ablation of epidermal RXRα in cooperation with activated CDK4 and oncogenic NRAS generates spontaneous and acute neonatal UVB induced malignant metastatic melanomas. BMC Cancer 2017;17(1):736.
114. Wang Z, Coleman DJ, Bajaj G, et al. RXRα ablation in epidermal keratinocytes enhances UVR-induced DNA damage, apoptosis, and proliferation of keratinocytes and melanocytes. J Invest Dermatol 2011;131(1):177–87.
115. Arnette CR, Roth-Carter QR, Koetsier JL, et al. Keratinocyte cadherin desmoglein 1 controls melanocyte behavior through paracrine signaling. Pigment Cell Melanoma Res 2020;33(2):305–17.
116. Faries MB, Thompson JF, Cochran AJ, et al. Completion Dissection or Observation for Sentinel-Node Metastasis in Melanoma. N Engl J Med 2017;376(23):2211–22.
117. Ulmer A, Schmidt-Kittler O, Fischer J, et al. Immunomagnetic enrichment, genomic characterization, and prognostic impact of circulating melanoma cells. Clin Cancer Res 2004;10(2):531–7.
118. MacKie RM, Reid R, Junor B. Fatal melanoma transferred in a donated kidney 16 years after melanoma surgery. N Engl J Med 2003;348(6):567–8.
119. Strauss DC, Thomas JM. Transmission of donor melanoma by organ transplantation. Lancet Oncol 2010;11(8):790–6.
120. Turner N, Ware O, Bosenberg M. Genetics of metastasis: melanoma and other cancers. Clin Exp Metastasis 2018;35(5–6):379–91.
121. Field MG, Durante MA, Anbunathan H, et al. Punctuated evolution of canonical genomic aberrations in uveal melanoma. Nat Commun 2018;9(1):116.
122. Harbour JW, Onken MD, Roberson ED, et al. Frequent mutation of BAP1 in metastasizing uveal melanomas. Science 2010;330(6009):1410–3.
123. Kim M, Gans JD, Nogueira C, et al. Comparative oncogenomics identifies NEDD9 as a melanoma metastasis gene. Cell 2006;125(7):1269–81.

124. Eroglu Z, Holmen SL, Chen Q, et al. Melanoma central nervous system metastases: An update to approaches, challenges, and opportunities. Pigment Cell Melanoma Res 2019;32(3):458–69.
125. Davies MA, Saiag P, Robert C, et al. Dabrafenib plus trametinib in patients with BRAF(V600)-mutant melanoma brain metastases (COMBI-MB): a multicentre, multicohort, open-label, phase 2 trial. Lancet Oncol 2017;18(7):863–73.
126. Tawbi HA, Forsyth PA, Algazi A, et al. Combined nivolumab and ipilimumab in melanoma metastatic to the brain. N Engl J Med 2018;379(8):722–30.
127. Fischer GM, Jalali A, Kircher DA, et al. Molecular profiling reveals unique immune and metabolic features of melanoma brain metastases. Cancer Discov 2019;9(5):628–45.
128. Cartlidge RA, Thomas GR, Cagnol S, et al. Oncogenic BRAF(V600E) inhibits BIM expression to promote melanoma cell survival. Pigment Cell Melanoma Res 2008;21(5):534–44.
129. Wang YF, Jiang CC, Kiejda KA, et al. Apoptosis induction in human melanoma cells by inhibition of MEK is caspase-independent and mediated by the Bcl-2 family members PUMA, Bim, and Mcl-1. Clin Cancer Res 2007;13(16):4934–42.
130. Montero J, Gstalder C, Kim DJ, et al. Destabilization of NOXA mRNA as a common resistance mechanism to targeted therapies. Nat Commun 2019;10(1): 5157.
131. Davies H, Bignell GR, Cox C, et al. Mutations of the BRAF gene in human cancer. Nature 2002;417(6892):949–94.
132. Satyamoorthy K, Li G, Gerrero MR, et al. Constitutive mitogen-activated protein kinase activation in melanoma is mediated by both BRAF mutations and autocrine growth factor stimulation. Cancer Res 2003;63(4):756–9.
133. Hingorani SR, Jacobetz MA, Robertson GP, et al. Suppression of BRAF(V599E) in human melanoma abrogates transformation. Cancer Res 2003;63(17): 5198–202.
134. Stadelmeyer E, Heitzer E, Resel M, et al. The BRAF V600K mutation is more frequent than the BRAF V600E mutation in melanoma in situ of lentigo maligna type. J Invest Dermatol 2014;134(2):548–50.
135. Menzies AM, Haydu LE, Visintin L, et al. Distinguishing clinicopathologic features of patients with V600E and V600K BRAF-mutant metastatic melanoma. Clin Cancer Res 2012;18(12):3242–9.
136. Hutchinson KE, Lipson D, Stephens PJ, et al. BRAF fusions define a distinct molecular subset of melanomas with potential sensitivity to MEK inhibition. Clin Cancer Res 2013;19(24):6696–702.
137. Turner JA, Bemis JGT, Bagby SM, et al. BRAF fusions identified in melanomas have variable treatment responses and phenotypes. Oncogene 2019;38(8): 1296–308.
138. Palanisamy N, Ateeq B, Kalyana-Sundaram S, et al. Rearrangements of the RAF kinase pathway in prostate cancer, gastric cancer and melanoma. Nat Med 2010;16(7):793–8.
139. Chapman PB, Hauschild A, Robert C, et al. Improved survival with vemurafenib in melanoma with BRAF V600E mutation. N Engl J Med 2011;364(26):2507–16.
140. Hauschild A, Grob JJ, Demidov LV, et al. Dabrafenib in BRAF-mutated metastatic melanoma: a multicentre, open-label, phase 3 randomised controlled trial. Lancet 2012;380(9839):358–65.
141. Dummer R, Ascierto PA, Gogas HJ, et al. Overall survival in patients with BRAF-mutant melanoma receiving encorafenib plus binimetinib versus vemurafenib or

encorafenib (COLUMBUS): a multicentre, open-label, randomised, phase 3 trial. Lancet Oncol 2018;19(10):1315–27.

142. Dahlman KB, Xia J, Hutchinson K, et al. BRAF(L597) mutations in melanoma are associated with sensitivity to MEK inhibitors. Cancer Discov 2012;2(9):791–7.

143. Falchook GS, Lewis KD, Infante JR, et al. Activity of the oral MEK inhibitor trametinib in patients with advanced melanoma: a phase 1 dose-escalation trial. Lancet Oncol 2012;13(8):782–9.

144. Ascierto PA, Schadendorf D, Berking C, et al. MEK162 for patients with advanced melanoma harbouring NRAS or Val600 BRAF mutations: a non-randomised, open-label phase 2 study. Lancet Oncol 2013;14(3):249–56.

145. Deuker MM, Marsh Durban V, Phillips WA, et al. PI3'-kinase inhibition forestalls the onset of MEK1/2 inhibitor resistance in BRAF-mutated melanoma. Cancer Discov 2015;5(2):143–53.

146. Kwong LN, Costello JC, Liu H, et al. Oncogenic NRAS signaling differentially regulates survival and proliferation in melanoma. Nat Med 2012;18(10):1503–10.

147. Sullivan RJ. Dual MAPK/CDK targeting in melanoma: new approaches, new challenges. Cancer Discov 2018;8(5):532–3.

148. Yin C, Zhu B, Zhang T, et al. Pharmacological targeting of STK19 inhibits oncogenic NRAS-driven melanomagenesis. Cell 2019;176(5):1113–27.e16.

149. Krauthammer M, Kong Y, Bacchiocchi A, et al. Exome sequencing identifies recurrent mutations in NF1 and RASopathy genes in sun-exposed melanomas. Nat Genet 2015;47(9):996–1002.

150. Nissan MH, Pratilas CA, Jones AM, et al. Loss of NF1 in cutaneous melanoma is associated with RAS activation and MEK dependence. Cancer Res 2014;74(8):2340–50.

151. Maertens O, Kuzmickas R, Manchester HE, et al. MAPK Pathway Suppression Unmasks Latent DNA Repair Defects and Confers a Chemical Synthetic Vulnerability in BRAF-, NRAS-, and NF1-Mutant Melanomas. Cancer Discov 2019;9(4):526–45.

152. Damsky W, Micevic G, Meeth K, et al. mTORC1 activation blocks BrafV600E-induced growth arrest but is insufficient for melanoma formation. Cancer Cell 2015;27(1):41–56.

153. Teh JLF, Cheng PF, Purwin TJ, et al. In In Vivo E2F reporting reveals efficacious schedules of MEK1/2-CDK4/6 Targeting and mTOR-S6 Resistance Mechanisms. Cancer Discov 2018;8(5):568–81.

154. Apostoli P, Minoia C, Hamilton EI. Significance and utility of reference values in occupational medicine. Sci Total Environ 1998;209(1):69–77.

155. Stambolic V, Suzuki A, de la Pompa JL, et al. Negative regulation of PKB/Akt-dependent cell survival by the tumor suppressor PTEN. Cell 1998;95(1):29–39.

156. Goel VK, Lazar AJ, Warneke CL, et al. Examination of mutations in BRAF, NRAS, and PTEN in primary cutaneous melanoma. J Invest Dermatol 2006;126(1):154–60.

157. Tsao H, Goel V, Wu H, et al. Genetic interaction between NRAS and BRAF mutations and PTEN/MMAC1 inactivation in melanoma. J Invest Dermatol 2004;122(2):337–41.

158. Mirmohammadsadegh A, Marini A, Nambiar S, et al. Epigenetic silencing of the PTEN gene in melanoma. Cancer Res 2006;66(13):6546–52.

159. Marsh Durban V, Deuker MM, Bosenberg MW, et al. Differential AKT dependency displayed by mouse models of BRAFV600E-initiated melanoma. J Clin Invest 2013;123(12):5104–18.

160. Nobes CD, Hall A. Rho, rac, and cdc42 GTPases regulate the assembly of multi-molecular focal complexes associated with actin stress fibers, lamellipodia, and filopodia. Cell 1995;81(1):53–62.

161. Krauthammer M, Kong Y, Ha BH, et al. Exome sequencing identifies recurrent somatic RAC1 mutations in melanoma. Nat Genet 2012;44(9):1006–14.

162. Hodis E, Watson IR, Kryukov GV, et al. A landscape of driver mutations in melanoma. Cell 2012;150(2):251–63.

163. Berger MF, Hodis E, Heffernan TP, et al. Melanoma genome sequencing reveals frequent PREX2 mutations. Nature 2012;485(7399):502–6.

164. Lionarons DA, Hancock DC, Rana S, et al. RAC1(P29S) induces a mesenchymal phenotypic switch via serum response factor to promote melanoma development and therapy resistance. Cancer Cell 2019;36(1):68–83.e9.

165. Lissauro Deribe Y, Shi Y, Rai K, et al. Truncating PREX2 mutations activate its GEF activity and alter gene expression regulation in NRAS-mutant melanoma. Proc Natl Acad Sci USA 2016;113(9):E1296–305.

166. Watson IR, Li L, Cabeceiras PK, et al. The RAC1 P29S hotspot mutation in melanoma confers resistance to pharmacological inhibition of RAF. Cancer Res 2014;74(17):4845–52.

167. Zeng H, Jorapur A, Shain AH, et al. Bi-allelic loss of CDKN2A initiates melanoma invasion via BRN2 activation. Cancer Cell 2018;34(1):56–68.e9.

168. McNeal AS, Liu K, Nakhate V, et al. CDKN2B loss promotes progression from benign melanocytic nevus to melanoma. Cancer Discov 2015;5(10):1072–85.

169. Mavrakis KJ, McDonald ER, Schlabach MR, et al. Disordered methionine metabolism in MTAP/CDKN2A-deleted cancers leads to dependence on PRMT5. Science 2016;351(6278):1208–13.

170. Marjon K, Cameron MJ, Quang P, et al. MTAP deletions in cancer create vulnerability to targeting of the MAT2A/PRMT5/RIOK1 Axis. Cell Rep 2016;15(3):574–87.

171. Huang FW, Hodis E, Xu MJ, et al. Highly recurrent TERT promoter mutations in human melanoma. Science 2013;339(6122):957–9.

172. Hayward NK, Wilmott JS, Waddell N, et al. Whole-genome landscapes of major melanoma subtypes. Nature 2017;545(7653):175–80.

173. Heidenreich B, Nagore E, Rachakonda PS, et al. Telomerase reverse transcriptase promoter mutations in primary cutaneous melanoma. Nat Commun 2014;5:3401.

174. Nagore E, Heidenreich B, Requena C, et al. TERT promoter mutations associate with fast-growing melanoma. Pigment Cell Melanoma Res 2016;29(2):236–8.

175. Osella-Abate S, Bertero L, Senetta R, et al. TERT promoter mutations are associated with visceral spreading in melanoma of the trunk. Cancers (Basel) 2019;11(4). https://doi.org/10.3390/cancers11040452.

176. Killela PJ, Reitman ZJ, Jiao Y, et al. TERT promoter mutations occur frequently in gliomas and a subset of tumors derived from cells with low rates of self-renewal. Proc Natl Acad Sci U S A 2013;110(15):6021–6.

177. Bai X, Kong Y, Chi Z, et al. MAPK Pathway and TERT promoter gene mutation pattern and its prognostic value in melanoma patients: a retrospective study of 2,793 cases. Clin Cancer Res 2017;23(20):6120–7.

178. Curtin JA, Busam K, Pinkel D, et al. Somatic activation of KIT in distinct subtypes of melanoma. J Clin Oncol 2006;24(26):4340–1.

179. Hemesath TJ, Price ER, Takemoto C, et al. MAP kinase links the transcription factor Microphthalmia to c-Kit signalling in melanocytes. Nature 1998;391(6664):298–301.

180. Van Raamsdonk CD, Bezrookove V, Green G, et al. Frequent somatic mutations of GNAQ in uveal melanoma and blue naevi. Nature 2009;457(7229):599–602.
181. Van Raamsdonk CD, Griewank KG, Crosby MB, et al. Mutations in GNA11 in uveal melanoma. N Engl J Med 2010;363(23):2191–9.
182. Moore AR, Ceraudo E, Sher JJ, et al. Recurrent activating mutations of G-protein-coupled receptor CYSLTR2 in uveal melanoma. Nat Genet 2016;48(6): 675–80.
183. Johansson P, Aoude LG, Wadt K, et al. Deep sequencing of uveal melanoma identifies a recurrent mutation in PLCB4. Oncotarget 2016;7(4):4624–31.
184. Robertson AG, Shih J, Yau C, et al. Integrative analysis identifies four molecular and clinical subsets in uveal melanoma. Cancer Cell 2017;32(2):204–20.e15.
185. Lian CG, Xu Y, Ceol C, et al. Loss of 5-hydroxymethylcytosine is an epigenetic hallmark of melanoma. Cell 2012;150(6):1135–46.
186. Ceol CJ, Houvras Y, Jane-Valbuena J, et al. The histone methyltransferase SETDB1 is recurrently amplified in melanoma and accelerates its onset. Nature 2011;471(7339):513–7.
187. Kato S, Yu Weng Q, Insco ML, et al. Gain-of-function genetic alterations of G9a drive oncogenesis. Cancer Discov 2020;10(7):980–97.
188. Lu C, Allis CD. SWI/SNF complex in cancer. Nat Genet 2017;49(2):178–9.
189. Shen J, Peng Y, Wei L, et al. ARID1A deficiency impairs the DNA damage checkpoint and sensitizes cells to PARP inhibitors. Cancer Discov 2015;5(7): 752–67.
190. Watanabe R, Ui A, Kanno S, et al. SWI/SNF factors required for cellular resistance to DNA damage include ARID1A and ARID1B and show interdependent protein stability. Cancer Res 2014;74(9):2465–75.
191. Mittal P, Roberts CWM. The SWI/SNF complex in cancer - biology, biomarkers and therapy. Nat Rev Clin Oncol 2020;17(7):435.
192. Sosman JA, Kim KB, Schuchter L, et al. Survival in BRAF V600-mutant advanced melanoma treated with vemurafenib. N Engl J Med 2012;366(8): 707–14.
193. Johnson DB, Menzies AM, Zimmer L, et al. Acquired BRAF inhibitor resistance: A multicenter meta-analysis of the spectrum and frequencies, clinical behaviour, and phenotypic associations of resistance mechanisms. Eur J Cancer 2015; 51(18):2792–9.
194. Rizos H, Menzies AM, Pupo GM, et al. BRAF inhibitor resistance mechanisms in metastatic melanoma: spectrum and clinical impact. Clin Cancer Res 2014; 20(7):1965–77.
195. Van Allen EM, Wagle N, Sucker A, et al. The genetic landscape of clinical resistance to RAF inhibition in metastatic melanoma. Cancer Discov 2014;4(1): 94–109.
196. Johnson DB, Childress MA, Chalmers ZR, et al. BRAF internal deletions and resistance to BRAF/MEK inhibitor therapy. Pigment Cell Melanoma Res 2018; 31(3):432–6.
197. Shi H, Moriceau G, Kong X, et al. Melanoma whole-exome sequencing identifies (V600E)B-RAF amplification-mediated acquired B-RAF inhibitor resistance. Nat Commun 2012;3:724.
198. Shi H, Hugo W, Kong X, et al. Acquired resistance and clonal evolution in melanoma during BRAF inhibitor therapy. Cancer Discov 2014;4(1):80–93.
199. Poulikakos PI, Persaud Y, Janakiraman M, et al. RAF inhibitor resistance is mediated by dimerization of aberrantly spliced BRAF(V600E). Nature 2011; 480(7377):387–90.

200. Ahronian LG, Sennott EM, Van Allen EM, et al. Clinical Acquired Resistance to RAF Inhibitor Combinations in BRAF-Mutant Colorectal Cancer through MAPK Pathway Alterations. Cancer Discov 2015;5(4):358–67.

201. Long GV, Fung C, Menzies AM, et al. Increased MAPK reactivation in early resistance to dabrafenib/trametinib combination therapy of BRAF-mutant metastatic melanoma. Nat Commun 2014;5:5694.

202. Moriceau G, Hugo W, Hong A, et al. Tunable-combinatorial mechanisms of acquired resistance limit the efficacy of BRAF/MEK cotargeting but result in melanoma drug addiction. Cancer Cell 2015;27(2):240–56.

203. Lu H, Liu S, Zhang G, et al. PAK signalling drives acquired drug resistance to MAPK inhibitors in BRAF-mutant melanomas. Nature 2017;550(7674):133–6.

204. Johannessen CM, Johnson LA, Piccioni F, et al. A melanocyte lineage program confers resistance to MAP kinase pathway inhibition. Nature 2013;504(7478): 138–42.

205. Smith MP, Brunton H, Rowling EJ, et al. Inhibiting drivers of non-mutational drug tolerance is a salvage strategy for targeted melanoma therapy. Cancer Cell 2016;29(3):270–84.

206. Tirosh I, Izar B, Prakadan SM, et al. Dissecting the multicellular ecosystem of metastatic melanoma by single-cell RNA-seq. Science 2016;352(6282):189–96.

207. Boshuizen J, Koopman LA, Krijgsman O, et al. Cooperative targeting of melanoma heterogeneity with an AXL antibody-drug conjugate and BRAF/MEK inhibitors. Nat Med 2018;24(2):203–12.

208. Hoek KS, Eichhoff OM, Schlegel NC, et al. In In vivo switching of human melanoma cells between proliferative and invasive states. Cancer Res 2008;68(3): 650–6.

209. Hoek KS, Schlegel NC, Brafford P, et al. Metastatic potential of melanomas defined by specific gene expression profiles with no BRAF signature. Pigment Cell Res 2006;19(4):290–302.

210. Verfaillie A, Imrichova H, Atak ZK, et al. Decoding the regulatory landscape of melanoma reveals TEADS as regulators of the invasive cell state. Nat Commun 2015;6:6683.

211. Konieczkowski DJ, Johannessen CM, Abudayyeh O, et al. A melanoma cell state distinction influences sensitivity to MAPK pathway inhibitors. Cancer Discov 2014;4(7):816–27.

212. Muller J, Krijgsman O, Tsoi J, et al. Low MITF/AXL ratio predicts early resistance to multiple targeted drugs in melanoma. Nat Commun 2014;5:5712.

213. Sensi M, Catani M, Castellano G, et al. Human cutaneous melanomas lacking MITF and melanocyte differentiation antigens express a functional Axl receptor kinase. J Invest Dermatol 2011;131(12):2448–57.

214. Ennen M, Keime C, Gambi G, et al. MITF-High and MITF-low cells and a novel subpopulation expressing genes of both cell states contribute to intra- and intertumoral heterogeneity of primary melanoma. Clin Cancer Res 2017;23(22): 7097–107.

215. Song C, Piva M, Sun L, et al. Recurrent tumor cell-intrinsic and -extrinsic alterations during MAPKi-induced melanoma regression and early adaptation. Cancer Discov 2017;7(11):1248–65.

216. Su Y, Wei W, Robert L, et al. Single-cell analysis resolves the cell state transition and signaling dynamics associated with melanoma drug-induced resistance. Proc Natl Acad Sci U S A 2017;114(52):13679–84.

217. Rambow F, Rogiers A, Marin-Bejar O, et al. Toward minimal residual disease-directed therapy in melanoma. Cell 2018;174(4):843–55.e19.

218. Tsoi J, Robert L, Paraiso K, et al. Multi-stage differentiation defines melanoma subtypes with differential vulnerability to drug-induced iron-dependent oxidative stress. Cancer Cell 2018;33(5):890–904.e5.
219. Young HL, Rowling EJ, Bugatti M, et al. An adaptive signaling network in melanoma inflammatory niches confers tolerance to MAPK signaling inhibition. J Exp Med 2017;214(6):1691–710.
220. Riesenberg S, Groetchen A, Siddaway R, et al. MITF and c-Jun antagonism interconnects melanoma dedifferentiation with pro-inflammatory cytokine responsiveness and myeloid cell recruitment. Nat Commun 2015;6:8755.
221. Smith MP, Sanchez-Laorden B, O'Brien K, et al. The immune microenvironment confers resistance to MAPK pathway inhibitors through macrophage-derived TNFα. Cancer Discov 2014;4(10):1214–29.
222. Kim IS, Heilmann S, Kansler ER, et al. Microenvironment-derived factors driving metastatic plasticity in melanoma. Nat Commun 2017;8:14343.
223. Kohler C, Nittner D, Rambow F, et al. Mouse cutaneous melanoma induced by mutant braf arises from expansion and dedifferentiation of mature pigmented melanocytes. Cell Stem Cell 2017;21(5):679–93.e6.
224. Wang L, Leite de Oliveira R, Huijberts S, et al. An acquired vulnerability of drug-resistant melanoma with therapeutic potential. Cell 2018;173(6):1413–25.e14.
225. Eggermont AMM, Blank CU, Mandala M, et al. Adjuvant pembrolizumab versus placebo in resected stage III melanoma. N Engl J Med 2018;378(19):1789–801.
226. Schoenfeld AJ, Hellmann MD. Acquired resistance to immune checkpoint inhibitors. Cancer Cell 2020;37(4):443–55.
227. Sade-Feldman M, Jiao YJ, Chen JH, et al. Resistance to checkpoint blockade therapy through inactivation of antigen presentation. Nat Commun 2017;8(1):1136.
228. Zaretsky JM, Garcia-Diaz A, Shin DS, et al. Mutations associated with acquired resistance to PD-1 blockade in melanoma. N Engl J Med 2016;375(9):819–29.
229. Liu D, Schilling B, Liu D, et al. Integrative molecular and clinical modeling of clinical outcomes to PD1 blockade in patients with metastatic melanoma. Nat Med 2019;25(12):1916–27.
230. Lee JH, Shklovskaya E, Yin Lim S, et al. Transcriptional downregulation of MHC class I and melanoma de- differentiation in resistance to PD-1 inhibition. Nat Commun 2020;11:1897. https://doi.org/10.1038/s41467-020-15726-7.
231. Hugo W, Shi H, Sun L, et al. Non-genomic and Immune Evolution of Melanoma Acquiring MAPKi Resistance. Cell 2015;162(6):1271–85.
232. Perez-Guijarro E, Yang HH, Araya RE, et al. Multimodel preclinical platform predicts clinical response of melanoma to immunotherapy. Nat Med 2020;26(5):781.
233. Mehta A, Kim YJ, Robert L, et al. Immunotherapy resistance by inflammation-induced dedifferentiation. Cancer Discov 2018;8(8):935–43.
234. Sade-Feldman M, Yizhak K, Bjorgaard SL, et al. Defining T cell states associated with response to checkpoint immunotherapy in melanoma. Cell 2018;175(4):998–1013.e20.
235. Jerby-Arnon L, Shah P, Cuoco MS, et al. A cancer cell program promotes T cell exclusion and resistance to checkpoint blockade. Cell 2018;175(4):984–97.e24.
236. Pan D, Kobayashi A, Jiang P, et al. A major chromatin regulator determines resistance of tumor cells to T cell-mediated killing. Science 2018;359(6377):770–5.

237. Zingg D, Arenas-Ramirez N, Sahin D, et al. The histone methyltransferase Ezh2 controls mechanisms of adaptive resistance to tumor immunotherapy. Cell Rep 2017;20(4):854–67.

238. Sheng W, LaFleur MW, Nguyen TH, et al. LSD1 ablation stimulates anti-tumor immunity and enables checkpoint blockade. Cell 2018;174(3):549–63.e19.

239. Li J, Wang W, Zhang Y, et al. Epigenetic driver mutations in ARID1A shape cancer immune phenotype and immunotherapy. J Clin Invest 2020;130(5):2712–26.

240. Goh G, Walradt T, Markarov V, et al. Mutational landscape of MCPyV-positive and MCPyV-negative Merkel cell carcinomas with implications for immunotherapy. Oncotarget 2016;7(3):3403–15.

241. Cimino PJ, Robirds DH, Tripp SR, et al. Retinoblastoma gene mutations detected by whole exome sequencing of Merkel cell carcinoma. Mod Pathol 2014;27(8):1073–87.

242. Bonilla X, Parmentier L, King B, et al. Genomic analysis identifies new drivers and progression pathways in skin basal cell carcinoma. Nat Genet 2016; 48(4):398–406.

243. Inman GJ, Wang J, Nagano A, et al. The genomic landscape of cutaneous SCC reveals drivers and a novel azathioprine associated mutational signature. Nat Commun 2018;9(1):3667.

244. Grossman RL, Heath AP, Ferretti V, et al. Toward a shared vision for cancer genomic data. N Engl J Med 2016;375(12):1109–12.

Epidemiology of Melanoma

Nicole L. Bolick, MD, MPH, MS[a,b], Alan C. Geller, MPH, RN[c],*

KEYWORDS

- Epidemiology • Melanoma • Public health • Screening

KEY POINTS

- Melanoma is a growing public health problem within the United States and across the world with incidence and mortality rates continuing to increase.
- Melanoma rates differ by geographic location, country, gender, age, occupation, and socioeconomic status.
- While population-based screening is not currently recommended, strategies to educate and screen high-risk individuals is of critical importance.
- While it appears that treatment is improving survival for Stage 4 patients, trying to understand the variables associated with those patients who receive therapy versus those who do not is essential.

INTRODUCTION

Melanoma is the most commonly fatal type of skin cancer and it is an important and growing public health problem in the United States, Australia, New Zealand, and Europe. Although incidence rates have been rising throughout the world for the past 5 decades, there have been some encouraging trends among the youngest populations in the United States and Australia. Concurrent with rising incidence trends, the mortality rate in most of the world had been rising as well, albeit slower than that for incidence. Only recently, likely due to the availability of new treatments for stage 4 melanoma, mortality rates in the United States dropped 18% from 2013 to 2016 (most recent year provided). Herein, we further describe trends in melanoma incidence and mortality, review the literature on risk factors, and provide an up-to-date assessment of population-wide screening.

[a] Harvard T.H. Chan School of Public Health, Kresge Building Room 718, 677 Huntington Ave, Boston, MA 02115, USA; [b] Department of Internal Medicine, East Carolina University/Vidant Medical Center, 600 Moye Boulevard, MA-350, Greenville, NC 27834, USA; [c] Department of Social and Behavioral Sciences, Harvard T.H. Chan School of Public Health, Kresge Building, Room 718, 677 Huntington Avenue, Boston, MA 02115, USA
* Corresponding author.
E-mail address: ageller@hsph.harvard.edu

Hematol Oncol Clin N Am 35 (2021) 57–72
https://doi.org/10.1016/j.hoc.2020.08.011
0889-8588/21/© 2020 Elsevier Inc. All rights reserved.

MELANOMA INCIDENCE AND MORTALITY RATES
Melanoma in the United States

Rates of melanoma continue to increase annually within the United States. In 2016 there were 82,476 new cases of melanoma reported.[1] The average annual percent change (AAPC) of melanoma age-adjusted incidence rates in non-Hispanic whites increased 2% from 2008 to 2017.[2] Approximately 7230 individuals died from melanoma in 2019 and if trends in melanoma death rates continue, melanoma is projected to be the only cancer objective to not meet the target for reduction in cancer deaths in Healthy People 2020.[3,4]

Incidence by Gender

Of additional concern is that the incidence of melanoma continues to increase with a greater change in incidence rate for men (**Fig. 1**).[2] From 2001 to 2017, age-adjusted incidence rates for melanoma in men of all races increased from 24.63 to 31.72 per 100,000 compared with an increase of 16.33 to 20.75 per 100,000 in women.[2] The melanoma incidence rate in men is increasing by 2.4% per year compared with a 1.7% increase in women.[5] These increasing melanoma incidence rates within the United States reflect the need for additional resources to combat rising melanoma rates.

Incidence by Age Group

Melanoma incidence rates vary among different age groups with data supporting statistically significant increases in melanoma rates from 2001 to 2015 for all age groups

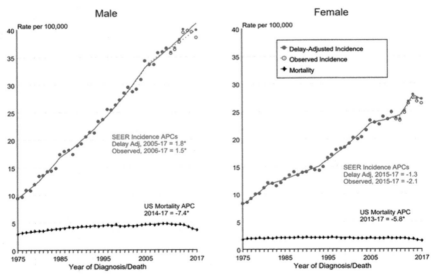

Fig. 1. SEER observed incidence, SEER delay adjusted incidence, and US death rates of melanoma of the skin, white, by sex. *The annual percent change is significantly different from zero (P<.05) *From* Howlader N, Noone AM, Krapcho M, Miller D, Brest A, Yu M, Ruhl J, Tatalovich Z, Mariotto A, Lewis DR, Chen HS, Feuer EJ, Cronin KA (eds). SEER Cancer Statistics Review, 1975-2017, National Cancer Institute. Bethesda, MD, https://seer.cancer.gov/csr/1975_2017/, based on November 2019 SEER data submission, posted to the SEER web site, April 2020.

35 years and older.[6] There has been a statistically significant decrease in melanoma rates from 2006 to 2015 for individuals ages 20 to 24 and 25 to 29 years.[6] For individuals ages 15 to 29 years there was a 3.6% annual decrease in melanoma rates for men (2004–2012) and a 3.3% annual decrease for women (2005–2012) reflecting a potential stabilization in this age group.[7] Most melanoma cases diagnosed between 2001 and 2015 were in adults who were 45 years and older (83.5%).[6] In white individuals younger than 60 years, melanoma rates are not projected to stabilize in the United States until 2021.[8]

Incidence Rates by Geography

Geographic differences in melanoma incidence rates across the United States exist (**Fig. 2**). From 2014 to 2015, 15 states had age-standardized incidence rates of melanoma that were greater than 30 per 100,000 individuals compared with only New Mexico and Hawaii from 2001 to 2002.[6] The 5 states with the greatest increase in age-standardized melanoma incidence rates from 2011 to 2015 from highest to lowest change were Maryland, Oklahoma, Indiana, Ohio, and Utah.[6] Alaska had the lowest

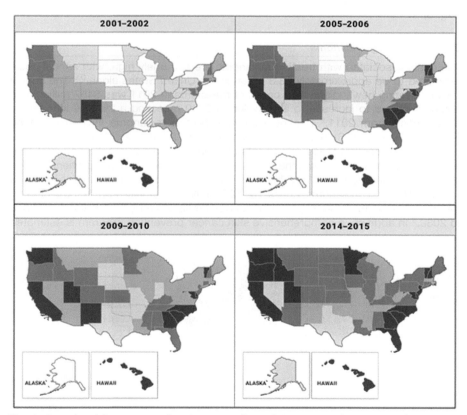

Fig. 2. State-level heat maps showing age-adjusted invasive melanoma incidence rates among non-Hispanic whites in 2001 to 2002, 2005 to 2006, 2009 to 2010, and 2014 to 2015. *From* Thrift AP, Gudenkauf FJ. Melanoma Incidence Among Non-Hispanic Whites in All 50 US States From 2001 Through 2015. *JNCI J Natl Cancer Inst.* Published online July 25, 2019:djz153. https://doi.org/10.1093/jnci/djz153

increase in age-adjusted incidence rates from 2011 to 2015.[6] These geographic differences reflect the need for additional research and public health campaigns in states with faster rising melanoma incidence rates to determine the reason for these rising rates.

Melanoma Mortality

From 2008 to 2017, the age-adjusted mortality rates decreased from 2.69 per 100,000 to 2.09 in the United States for all races and genders.[2] In 2017, age-adjusted mortality rates for melanoma were 2.09 per 100,000 for all races with a rate of 2.44 per 100,000 for whites.[2] The mortality rate for men is more than double that for women (3.59 per 100,000 for white men in 2017 compared with 1.52 per 100,000 in white women).[2] Comparable to other countries, the United States continues to see a greater mortality rate in older individuals, with those 85 or older having the highest age-specific mortality rate of 23.6 per 100,000 for all races and genders.[2] Melanoma mortality rates increase in the United States as individuals age, with men having greater mortality than women across almost all age groups.[2] Men comprised 59.3% of all cases and 65.6% of all deaths in 2019.[4] Melanoma mortality rates also differ among states (**Fig. 3**).[2]

Costs of Treating Melanoma

The costs associated with treating melanoma are extremely high, with annual costs estimated to be approximately $3.3 billion in the United States alone.[3,9] The annual cost of treating newly diagnosed cases of melanoma in 2011 was $457 million with costs estimated to increase to $1.6 billion in 2030 reflecting a 252.4% increase in annual costs from 2011.[9] Recent algorithms predict melanoma incidence among whites in the United States will peak from 2022 to 2026.[8] Additional interventions are needed to combat these rising costs of melanoma to prevent the potential economic burden associated with the disease. Implementation of a comprehensive skin cancer prevention program has been estimated to decrease the average costs of newly diagnosed melanoma cases by $250 million annually and is projected to decrease the costs of treating newly diagnosed melanoma by $2.7 billion from 2020 to 2030.[9] In addition, a comprehensive skin cancer prevention program is estimated

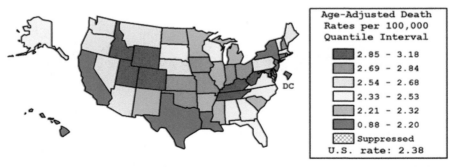

Fig. 3. Age-adjusted cancer death rates by state, all races, 2013 to 2017. *From* Howlader N, Noone AM, Krapcho M, Miller D, Brest A, Yu M, Ruhl J, Tatalovich Z, Mariotto A, Lewis DR, Chen HS, Feuer EJ, Cronin KA (eds). SEER Cancer Statistics Review, 1975-2017, National Cancer Institute. Bethesda, MD, https://seer.cancer.gov/csr/1975_2017/, based on November 2019 SEER data submission, posted to the SEER web site, April 2020.

to prevent approximately 230,000 cases of melanoma from 2020 to 2030 (20% of projected cases), which is approximately 21,000 cases of melanoma prevented per year.[9]

MELANOMA ACROSS THE WORLD
Incidence and Mortality

Melanoma incidence rates and mortality vary sharply across the world with 351,880 global cases of melanoma (2015) and 62,000 deaths from melanoma in 2015.[10] The number of cases grew from 232,000 in 2012 to 351,880 in 2015, although this could be related in part to improvements in cancer registration.[10,11] From 2006 to 2016, melanoma incidence increased 39% across the world with melanoma mortality rates estimated to account for 0.7% of deaths from all cancers.[11,12]

New Zealand, Australia, Norway, Sweden, and the Netherlands were the 5 countries in 2015 with the highest age-standardized melanoma incidence and mortality rates.[10] Melanoma mortality rates are highest in Australia and New Zealand, with both countries averaging an annual increase in melanoma mortality rates of 1.5% per year from 2001 to 2011.[8,10] In Queensland, Australia, from 2010 to 2014 the annual melanoma age-standardized mortality rate was 7 per 100,000 individuals.[13] Norway and Sweden had the highest melanoma mortality rates of all countries in the northern hemisphere and have been experiencing a small to modest increase in age-standardized melanoma mortality rates for several decades.[8] According to the most recent Globocan 2008 data, melanoma mortality is highest in Australia/New Zealand (3.5 per 100,000), North America (1.7 per 100,000), and Europe (1.5 per 100,000).[14]

Melanoma incidence rates have peaked at different time points across the world. Australia's melanoma incidence rates peaked around 2005 with future melanoma rates predicted to decline.[8] Melanoma incidence rates among younger individuals in Australia have started to stabilize, reflecting the possible success of public health prevention campaigns focusing on the importance of reducing sun exposure.[13,15] New Zealand's melanoma incidence rates are projected to peak between the time period of 2012 to 2016 and then are projected to decline in a similar trend to Australia.[8] Norway, Sweden, and the United Kingdom have all seen a greater than 3% annual increase in melanoma rates from 1982 to 2011 with rates projected to continue to rise until at least 2022.[8] In individuals younger than 60 years, melanoma rates are projected to not stabilize until 2026 for Norway, the United Kingdom, and Sweden.[8]

Worldwide Incidence by Gender

Men and women experience differences in disability-adjusted life years (DALYs) and melanoma mortality rates across the world. DALY rates were greater for men in 2015 across all world regions except for the regions of Western, Eastern, and Central sub-Saharan Africa (**Fig. 4**).[10] Global age-standardized melanoma DALY rates were 27 in men and 19 in women with melanoma leading to 1,596,262 worldwide DALYs in 2015 (**Fig. 5**).[10] The 5 countries with the highest age-standardized DALY rates in 2015 were New Zealand, Australia, Norway, the Netherlands, and Sweden.[10] Global melanoma mortality rates in 2015 followed a similar trend to DALY rates with men having higher mortality rates than women in most countries (**Fig. 6**).[10]

Worldwide Incidence by Age Group

In the United Kingdom, Norway, Sweden, New Zealand, Australia, and the United States, melanoma rates are highest for those older than 80 years, reflecting an unequal burden of melanoma in older populations.[8] In Queensland, Australia, from 1995 to 2014 there was only an increase in age-standardized incidence of invasive melanoma

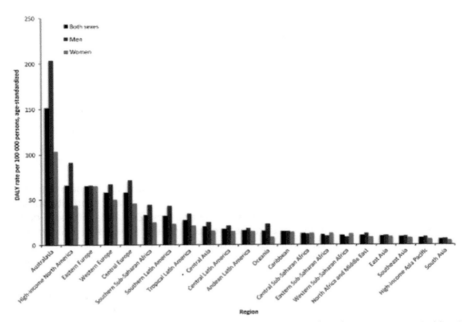

Fig. 4. Age-standardized melanoma DALY rates in 21 world regions by sex. *From* Karimkhani C, Green AC, Nijsten T, et al. The global burden of melanoma: results from the Global Burden of Disease Study 2015. *Br J Dermatol*. 2017;177(1):134-140. https://doi.org/10.1111/bjd.15510

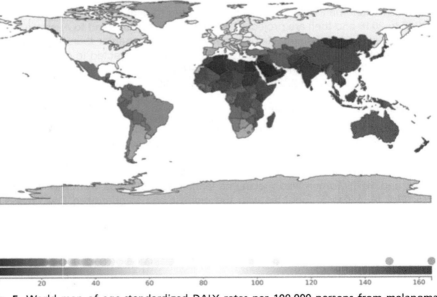

Fig. 5. World map of age-standardized DALY rates per 100,000 persons from melanoma, both sexes. *From* Karimkhani C, Green AC, Nijsten T, et al. The global burden of melanoma: results from the Global Burden of Disease Study 2015. *Br J Dermatol*. 2017;177(1):134-140. https://doi.org/10.1111/bjd.15510

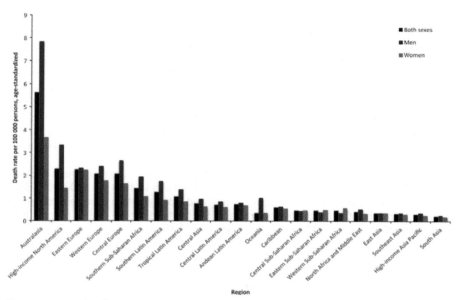

Fig. 6. Age-standardized melanoma mortality rates in 21 world regions by sex. *From* Karimkhani C, Green AC, Nijsten T, et al. The global burden of melanoma: results from the Global Burden of Disease Study 2015. *Br J Dermatol.* 2017;177(1):134-140. https://doi.org/10.1111/bjd.15510

in individuals 60 years or older with a deceleration in incidence rates over the 20-year study period.[13] Furthermore, differences in mortality exist for older individuals. For example, in Spain from 1975 to 2016, the melanoma mortality rates increased for those 69 years or older, while individuals younger than 50 experienced a decrease in mortality and those 50 to 59 years of age experienced a leveling off for mortality.[16] Increased mortality in older individuals is likely due to comorbidities, more advanced disease, and less robust immune systems.[16] Additional resources are needed in Europe, Australia, and the United States to combat the disparities in melanoma incidence and mortality rates across age groups.

Melanoma in Europe

Melanoma incidence began to increase shortly after World War II in Western countries and Europe.[17] Europe continues to have experience rising rates of melanoma with most countries experiencing a doubling of incidence rates from 1990 to 2005, with annual increases varying between 2% and 10%.[17] For example, in Germany from 1999 to 2012, age-standardized incidence rates (ASIRs) increased by 3% per year.[17] As with the United States, Germany continues to see a greater change in incidence rate for men with crude incidence rates increasing 4.8% annually for men from 1999 to 2012 and 3.9% annually for women during the same time period.[17] In addition, from 1995 to 2012 a recent study analyzing 117 million Europeans across 18 cancer registries in 13 countries showed a statistically significant increase for both invasive and in situ melanoma incidence across both genders.[18]

Europe has the third highest melanoma mortality rate across the world with men having higher mortality rates within the continent, likely because of worse survival.[14,18] Slovenia, Germany, the United Kingdom, and Ireland each had higher melanoma mortality rates in men especially during the time period of 1995 to 2012.[14,18] Countries within Central and Eastern Europe report lower survival and greater advanced tumor rates than other European countries and are estimated to experience the greatest percentage (35.5%) of the 20,000 melanoma deaths estimated to occur annually in Europe.[14] In 2012, there were approximately 100,000 new cases of melanoma in Europe with Central and Eastern Europe having 19% of these cases.[19] In South-Eastern Europe, melanoma incidence rates were uniformly increasing until 2010, especially in individuals older than 50 years.[19] Persistent differences in stabilization of mortality trends exist between Northwestern Europe and South-Eastern Europe reflecting the disparities in melanoma detection time between the 2 geographic regions.[19]

Within Europe, the highest reported melanoma incidence rates have been in Scandinavia with ASIRs ranging from 18 per 100,000 in Norway to 12.8 per 100,000 in Sweden.[17] These countries are followed by Central and Northwestern European countries such as Germany, the United Kingdom, and Switzerland where ASIRs ranged from 12.5 per to 28.7 per 100,000 individuals annnually.[17] The lowest ASIRs were reported in Mediterranean countries which may be due to inadequate recording of cancers or because of a lower percentage of lighter-skinned individuals.[17] Melanoma mortality rates from 1995 to 2012 showed an increase in rates in Northern Europe, with Iceland, Ireland, and Norway having rising AAPC (5.4%, 3.4% and 1.6%, respectively) (**Fig. 7**).[18]

In Europe, a study calculating regional average mortality-to-incidence ratios (MIR) using Globocan 2008 data concluded the average MIR was 0.13 in Western Europe,

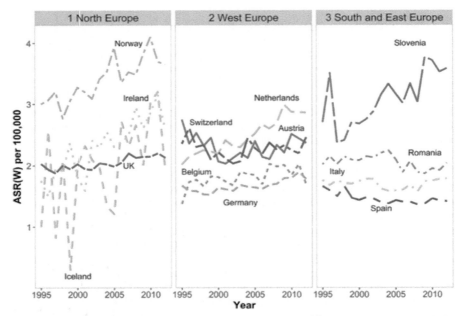

Fig. 7. Skin cancer mortality, 1995 to 2012. Both sexes. World age-standardized mortality trends for melanoma lesions in different European countries in the period 1995 to 2012. Data retrieved from the World Health Organizatoin mortality database. *From* Sacchetto L, Zanetti R, Comber H, et al. Trends in incidence of thick, thin and in situ melanoma in Europe. *Eur J Cancer.* 2018;92:108-118. https://doi.org/10.1016/j.ejca.2017.12.024

0.16 in Northern Europe, 0.2 in Southern Europe, and 0.35 in Eastern and Central Europe.[20] The investigators found significant inverse correlation ($P<.05$, $r = -0.76$) between the individual nation's melanoma MIR and health expenditure per capita for European countries.[20] There are geographic differences in melanoma rates across Europe with MIRs ranging from 0.09 in Switzerland to 0.44 in Latvia.[20] However, population-based cancer registries throughout Europe only provide information on approximately a third of Europe's population with several countries in Eastern and Central Europe lacking adequate cancer registration data.[20] There is a future need for more comprehensive population-based cancer data throughout Europe to best determine melanoma rates within the continent.

Melanoma in China

A recent, novel study analyzing the burden of melanoma in China concluded that the ASIRs of melanoma increased 0.6% annually from 1990 to 2005 and 6.1% from 2005 to 2017.[21] During this time period, the number of cases in China was 16,073 and the number of deaths was 5088.[21] From 1990 to 2017, the age-standardized incidence rate of melanoma increased 110.3% in China.[21] The age-standardized mortality rate decreased by an average of 1.6% annually from 1990 to 2006 and increased an average of 1.3% annually from 2006 to 2017 possibly reflecting the substantial increase in melanoma incidence rates beginning in 2005.[21]

RISK FACTORS

Intermittent sun exposure and sunburn history are both risk factors for the development of melanoma with approximately 80% of melanomas developing in locations that receive intermittent sun exposure.[15] Additional research continues to support a correlation of melanoma risk in those who began indoor tanning when younger than 25 years, with a sixfold increased risk in women younger than 30 years, a 3.5-fold increased risk for women 30 to 39 years, and a 2.3-fold increased risk in women 40 to 49 years.[22,23] With the addition of each primary melanoma, the odds of an individual ever having indoor tanned increases by 48%.[22,24] However, a recent study in Austria concluded that the development of subsequent melanomas after diagnosis of a first melanoma is most impacted by genetic variants, family history, actinic damage on the back, as well as number as nevi.[22,25]

Further investigation into lifestyle differences in melanoma risk need to be examined. A recent study concluded that alcohol use may be moderately associated with an increased risk of melanoma with additional research needed on this topic.[26,27] A recent case-control study concluded there is an association of vitamin D insufficiency/deficiency and melanoma as 66.2% of melanoma patients had vitamin D deficiency at the time of diagnosis and only 15.2% of non-melanoma patients were deficient.[28] Body mass may play a role in melanoma development with overweight individuals (body mass index ≥ 25) having a significantly increased melanoma risk in those less than 50 years of age (odds ratio [OR] 1.85) although the number of moles can be an important confounder.[29] Furthermore, in European populations recent traumatic events such as death of relative or personal major illness have been reported to be associated with increased melanoma risk (OR 3.41, $P<.05$).[27]

Patient's receiving psoralen and ultraviolet A (PUVA) treatment for skin conditions such as psoriasis are at increased risk of developing melanoma after 250 treatments.[30] In post-menopausal women aspirin use is associated with a lower risk of melanoma (21%) when compared with nonsteroidal anti-inflammatory drug nonusers, with a longer duration of aspirin use providing even more protection against melanoma.[31]

Socioeconomic status affects melanoma detection and disease outcome with individuals without insurance having a 67% greater risk of dying from melanoma than those with private insurance.[30] Furthermore, patients with Medicaid and Medicare have worse melanoma disease outcomes than individuals with private insurance.[30]

HOST FACTORS

The risk of melanoma varies greatly by race with a lifetime risk of 0.58% for Hispanic individuals, 0.1% for African American individuals, and 2.6% for Caucasians.[30] Compared with individuals with dark skin pigmentation, Caucasians are at an approximately 10-fold risk of melanoma.[30] According to some, any individual with at least one atypical nevi should have screening from every 3 months to once a year depending on their nevi characteristics as at least one atypical nevi is associated with a 2 to 15 increased fold risk of developing melanoma.[32,33] An especially high-risk group for developing melanoma is individuals with more than 25 nevi with 42% of melanomas being attributable to individuals with this risk factor.[32] Individuals with 11 to 25 nevi have 1.5 times higher risk of developing melanoma with this risk doubling with each additional increase of 25 nevi.[30]

Preexisting conditions such as irritable bowel disease (IBD), Parkinson disease, and history of childhood cancer are associated with higher melanoma risk.[34–36] Individuals with IBD are at an increased risk of developing melanoma with those with Crohn's disease having the greatest risk.[34] In addition, melanoma risk has been reported to be higher in individuals with Parkinson disease.[35] Adult survivors of childhood cancer may also have an increased risk of melanoma with data indicating that these individuals have a 2.5-fold increased risk.[36]

ENVIRONMENTAL RISK FACTORS

Recent studies have concluded that the melanoma MIR can be influenced by both sociodemographic and health care differences and these factors are able to predict how MIRs vary across geographic regions within the United States.[37] Using data from the 50 US states (1999-2014), percentage of non-Hispanic white individuals and number of active physicians were the two variables most strongly associated with MIR.[37] Intrinsic differences or the factors that states have in common were estimated to be associated with 99% of the variance in MIR between states suggesting that future interventions and policies designed to reduce melanoma rates may be more impactful at the state level than with a national focus.[37]

Multiple occupational exposures are associated with melanoma development including ultraviolet (UV) radiation from both welding fumes and arc welding.[30] The UV radiation exposure in welding has been shown to be correlated with the development of ocular melanoma with a prior study concluding French welders were at a 7.3 increased odds of developing ocular melanoma compared with the general French population.[30] Chronic exposure to UV light is associated with melanoma with an individual who has over 20 years of occupational sun exposure being at an increased risk for the development of melanoma.[30]

Occupational type can also lead to differences in the risk of developing melanoma. A recent metanalysis concluded that individuals in the oil/petroleum industries have a slightly increased melanoma incidence.[38] Men in the oil/petroleum industries and chemical industry workers have an increased melanoma mortality rate compared with the general population.[38] This may be due to confounding factors of sun exposure habits, worse melanoma survival among men, and exposure to pollutants.[38] Electrical industry workers were found to have a similar melanoma incidence and mortality rates to the general population.[38] Furthermore, exposure to pesticides has been shown to be significantly associated with melanoma risk with a recent meta-analysis concluding there is an increased melanoma risk after each use of a herbicide (summary relative risk of 1.85).[39] However, independently of the level of exposure neither pesticides in general nor insecticides were shown to be associated with greater melanoma risk.[39]

SCREENING FOR MELANOMA

The US Preventive Services Task Force concludes that the current evidence is insufficient and that the balance of benefits and harms of visual skin examination by a clinician to screen for skin cancer in asymptomatic adults cannot be determined. We review the relevant studies that have been conducted over the past decade.

Randomized trials have not been conducted for population-wide melanoma screening, and without data from randomized trials it is not clear that population-based screening will result in decreased mortality.[40,41] Herein, we use data from observational studies acknowledging the many limitations of using such data (lead time bias, length bias). At this point, it is highly unlikely that one will conduct a randomized trial as the current funding climate precludes a trial that would likely cost more than $70 million and it has been estimated that approximately 800,000 participants would be required to detect a difference in mortality because of the relatively low melanoma mortality rate.[41]

The benefits of screening for melanoma should be obvious because the prognosis of melanoma is so strongly associated with stage and thickness but there are many challenges. Detection by screening has been associated with thinner melanomas at diagnosis, prognosis is significantly better for thinner (early-stage) compared with later-stage melanoma, cutaneous melanoma is usually visible on the skin, visual skin examination is safe and well tolerated by patients, and risk factors for melanoma are readily identifiable.[40,41]

There are a number of limitations. First, it is unclear how many nondermatologist physicians are adequately trained in the skin cancer examination or have the time to perform a full-body skin examination including the back which makes up 30% of melanomas in men. Some melanomas may not be predisposed to early detection, particularly nodular melanoma, acral lentiginous melanoma, and desmoplastic melanoma. Although one does not have definitive data on this, screening may result in overdiagnosis of melanoma often because it is so slow-growing that it would most likely never have a significant impact on the patient during their lifetime.

The most far reaching observational trial for skin cancer screening took place first in Schleswig-Holstein, a northern state in Germany. This so-called pilot study, if successful, was to lead to a nationwide screening study in Germany. The SCREEN study started with a communications program to alert the public about the need for screening coupled with a training program of nondermatologist physicians led by dermatologists. More than 1600 physicians received 8 hours of training before screening and they were permitted to charge 25 Euros per examination. In all, 360,288 patients were screened (from an eligible population of 1.9 million), and 585 melanomas were detected. Screening took place between July 1, 2003, and June 30, 2004. Mortality data from Schleswig-Holstein was compared with neighboring states and Denmark and revealed a 47% mortality decline in men and 49% in women. Overall, 620 persons needed to be screened to detect 1 melanoma. Ninety percent of melanomas detected by screening were less than 1 mm thick. Five years following the screening effort, despite a screening participation rate less than 20%, mortality from melanoma among adults in the pilot program area was nearly 50% lower than in the rest of Germany and was lower than expected based on historical rates. However, the mortality decline seen at the 5-year mark was not sustained; 2 years later, mortality rates returned to the prescreening level.[42–46] While it was not sustained, the reasons for this are unclear although the national effort did not have a prescreening communication campaign such as the one in Schleswig-Holstein.

A population-based case-control study in Queensland, Australia, found that when compared with unscreened patients, primary care clinician screening was associated with thinner melanoma lesions. Full skin examinations by a clinician 3 years before diagnosis were associated with thinner melanomas compared with those who had not had a skin examination conferring a 14% lower risk for a melanoma greater than 0.75 mm thick. The decrease in risk was sharpest for the thickest melanomas (risk reduction 40% for lesions $\geq$3 mm).[47] In the Western Pennsylvania primary care physician-based screening intervention, clinician screening was associated with a higher rate of melanoma diagnoses, including increased diagnoses of stage T1 ($\leq$1 mm) melanoma and melanomas in situ, but not thicker melanomas.[48] A workplace time series conducted in northern California from 1965 to 1996, involving a comprehensive initiative of pre-awareness, education, and skin screening program, led to a reduction in the incidence of thicker melanoma and a lower-than-expected death rate compared with the statewide cancer registry statistics over the time period assessed.[49]

The value of clinician training to detect melanoma has been demonstrated in several studies. Most medical professionals lack specific education in early detection of melanoma. In a population-based screening program in the United States, the rate of melanoma diagnosis rose almost 80% among patients screened at practices with the highest proportion of providers trained using INFORMED (INternet curriculum FOR Melanoma Early Detection), an online educational system for primary care clinicians.[50–52]

A promising approach includes lesion-directed screening, in which clinicians evaluate lesions identified by patients using preselected criteria, required less time and resulted in similar melanoma detection rates as total skin examination in a study that assessed total body examination by experienced dermatologists in 2 sociodemographically similar regions in Belgium. Lesion-directed screening found a similar detection rate (2.3 vs 3.2%) but was notably 5.6 times less time-consuming.[53]

Screening for melanoma may save lives but may also cause patient distress. Risica and colleagues[54] investigated potential psychological harms and benefits of skin examinations by conducting telephone surveys in 2015 of 187 screened participants in the Western Pennsylvania study; all were $\geq$35 years old. Participants had their skin examined by practitioners who had completed INFORMED. Participants completed the Spielberger State-Trait Anxiety Inventory, Psychological Consequences of Screening (PCQ), Hospital Anxiety and Depression scale, and the 12-Item Short Form Health Survey (SF-12). Participants who were thoroughly screened did not differ on negative psychosocial measures; scored higher on measures of positive psychosocial well-being (PCQ); and were more motivated to conduct monthly self-examinations and seek annual clinician skin examinations, compared with other participants ($P<.05$). Importantly, post-screening, thoroughly screened patients were more likely to report skin prevention practices (skin self-examinations to identify a concerning lesion, practitioner provided skin examination), recommend skin examinations to peers, and feel satisfied with their skin cancer education than less thoroughly screened individuals ($P<.01$).[54]

Newer screening technologies might soon become available. Deep learning convolutional neural networks (CNNs) show potential for melanoma diagnosis. Melanoma thickness at diagnosis among others depends on melanoma localization and subtype (eg, advanced thickness in acro-lentiginous or nodular melanomas). The question whether CNN may counterbalance physicians' diagnostic difficulties in these melanomas has not been addressed. The CNN showed a high-level performance in set-SSM, set-NM and set-LMM (sensitivities >93.3%, specificities >65%, receiver operating characteristics-area under the curve >0.926).[55] In a separate study, Esteva and colleagues[56] demonstrated classification of skin lesions using a single CNN, trained end-to-end from images directly, using only pixels and disease labels as inputs. They tested its performance against 21 board-certified dermatologists on biopsy-proven clinical images with 2 critical binary classification use cases: keratinocyte carcinomas versus benign seborrheic keratoses; and cutaneous melanomas versus benign nevi. The CNN achieved performance equal to all tested experts across both tasks, demonstrating an artificial intelligence capable of classifying skin cancer with a level of competence comparable to dermatologists.[56]

ACKNOWLEDGMENTS

Author Contributions: Bolick and Geller had full access to all the data in the study and take responsibility for the integrity of the data and the accuracy of the data analysis. Study concept and design: Bolick and Geller. Acquisition, analysis, and interpretation of data: Bolick and Geller. Drafting of article and revising critically for important intellectual content: Bolick and Geller.

DISCLOSURE

The authors have nothing to disclosure.

REFERENCES

1. US Cancer Statistics Working Group, US Cancer. Statistics data visualizations tool, based on November 2018 submission data (1999-2016). Bethesda: US Department of Health and Human Services, Centers for Disease Control and Prevention and National Cancer Institute; 2019. Available at: www.cdc.gov/cancer/dataviz.
2. Howlader N, Noone AM, Krapcho M, et al, editors. SEER cancer statistics review, 1975-2017. Bethesda (MD): National Cancer Institute; 2020. based on November 2019 SEER data submission, posted to the SEER web site. Available at: https://seer.cancer.gov/csr/1975_2017/.
3. Koh HK, U.S. Department of Health and Human Services. The Surgeon General's call to action to prevent skin cancer. Washington, DC: U.S. Dept of Health and Human Services, Office of the Surgeon General; 2014. p. 112.
4. Street W, American Cancer Society. Cancer facts & figures 2019. Atlanta (GA): American Cancer Society; 2019.
5. Rahib L, Smith BD, Aizenberg R, et al. Projecting cancer incidence and deaths to 2030: the unexpected burden of thyroid, liver, and pancreas cancers in the United States. Cancer Res 2014;74(11):2913–21.
6. Thrift AP, Gudenkauf FJ. Melanoma incidence among non-Hispanic Whites in all 50 US states from 2001 through 2015. J Natl Cancer Inst 2019;djz153. https://doi.org/10.1093/jnci/djz153.
7. Watson M, Geller AC, Tucker MA, et al. Melanoma burden and recent trends among non-Hispanic whites aged 15–49 years, United States. Prev Med 2016; 91:294–8.

8. Whiteman DC, Green AC, Olsen CM. The growing burden of invasive melanoma: projections of incidence rates and numbers of new cases in six susceptible populations through 2031. J Invest Dermatol 2016;136(6):1161–71.

9. Guy GP Jr, Thomas CC, Thompson T, et al. Vital signs: melanoma incidence and mortality trends and projections - United States, 1982-2030. MMWR Morb Mortal Wkly Rep 2015;64(21):591–6.

10. Karimkhani C, Green AC, Nijsten T, et al. The global burden of melanoma: results from the Global Burden of Disease Study 2015. Br J Dermatol 2017;177(1): 134–40.

11. Dimitriou F, Krattinger R, Ramelyte E, et al. The world of melanoma: epidemiologic, genetic, and anatomic differences of melanoma across the globe. Curr Oncol Rep 2018;20(11):87.

12. Fitzmaurice C, Global Burden of Disease Cancer Collaboration. Global, regional, and national cancer incidence, mortality, years of life lost, years lived with disability, and disability-adjusted life-years for 29 cancer groups, 2006 to 2016: A systematic analysis for the Global Burden of Disease study. J Clin Oncol 2018;36(15_suppl):1568.

13. Aitken JF, Youlden DR, Baade PD, et al. Generational shift in melanoma incidence and mortality in Queensland, Australia, 1995-2014: Generational shift in melanoma. Int J Cancer 2018;142(8):1528–35.

14. Forsea AM, del Marmol V, de Vries E, et al. Melanoma incidence and mortality in Europe: new estimates, persistent disparities: Melanoma incidence and mortality disparities in Europe. Br J Dermatol 2012;167(5):1124–30.

15. Garbe C, Leiter U. Melanoma epidemiology and trends. Clin Dermatol 2009; 27(1):3–9.

16. Cayuela A, Cayuela L, Rodríguez-Domínguez S, et al. Is melanoma mortality declining in Spain? Analysis of trends from 1975 to 2016. Br J Dermatol 2018; 179(4):991–2.

17. Garbe C, Keim U, Eigentler TK, et al. Time trends in incidence and mortality of cutaneous melanoma in Germany. J Eur Acad Dermatol Venereol 2019;33(7): 1272–80.

18. Sacchetto L, Zanetti R, Comber H, et al. Trends in incidence of thick, thin and in situ melanoma in Europe. Eur J Cancer 2018;92:108–18.

19. Barbaric J, Sekerija M, Agius D, et al. Disparities in melanoma incidence and mortality in South-Eastern Europe: Increasing incidence and divergent mortality patterns. Is progress around the corner? Eur J Cancer 2016;55:47–55.

20. Forsea AM, del Marmol V, Stratigos A, et al. Melanoma prognosis in Europe: far from equal. Br J Dermatol 2014;171(1):179–82.

21. Wu Y, Wang Y, Wang L, et al. Burden of melanoma in China, 1990–2017: Findings from the 2017 global burden of disease study. Int J Cancer 2019. https://doi.org/10.1002/ijc.32764.

22. Suppa M, Gandini S. Sunbeds and melanoma risk: time to close the debate. Curr Opin Oncol 2019;31(2):65–71.

23. Lazovich D, Isaksson Vogel R, Weinstock MA, et al. Association between indoor tanning and melanoma in younger men and women. JAMA Dermatol 2016; 152(3):268.

24. Li Y, Kulkarni M, Trinkaus K, et al. Second primary melanomas: Increased risk and decreased time to presentation in patients exposed to tanning beds. J Am Acad Dermatol 2018;79(6):1101–8.

25. Müller C, Wendt J, Rauscher S, et al. Risk factors of subsequent primary melanomas in Austria. JAMA Dermatol 2019;155(2):188.

26. Gandini S, Masala G, Palli D, et al. Alcohol, alcoholic beverages, and melanoma risk: a systematic literature review and dose–response meta-analysis. Eur J Nutr 2018;57(7):2323–32.
27. de Vries E, Trakatelli M, Kalabalikis D, et al. Known and potential new risk factors for skin cancer in European populations: a multicentre case-control study: Risk factors for skin cancer in European populations. Br J Dermatol 2012;167:1–13.
28. Cattaruzza MS, Pisani D, Fidanza L, et al. 25-Hydroxyvitamin D serum levels and melanoma risk: a case–control study and evidence synthesis of clinical epidemiological studies. Eur J Cancer Prev 2019;28(3):203–11.
29. De Giorgi V, Gori A, Savarese I, et al. Role of BMI and hormone therapy in melanoma risk: a case–control study. J Cancer Res Clin Oncol 2017;143(7):1191–7.
30. Carr S, Smith C, Wernberg J. Epidemiology and risk factors of melanoma. Surg Clin North Am 2020;100(1):1–12.
31. Gamba CA, Swetter SM, Stefanick ML, et al. Aspirin is associated with lower melanoma risk among postmenopausal Caucasian women: The Women's Health Initiative. Cancer 2013;119(8):1562–9.
32. Mayer JE, Swetter SM, Fu T, et al. Screening, early detection, education, and trends for melanoma: Current status (2007-2013) and future directions. J Am Acad Dermatol 2014;71(4):611.e1-10.
33. Choi JN, Hanlon A, Leffell D. Melanoma and nevi: detection and diagnosis. Curr Probl Cancer 2011;35(4):138–61.
34. Long MD, Martin CF, Pipkin CA, et al. Risk of melanoma and nonmelanoma skin cancer among patients with inflammatory bowel disease. Gastroenterology 2012;143(2):390–9.e1.
35. Increased melanoma risk in Parkinson disease: a prospective clinicopathological study. Arch Neurol 2010;67(3):6.
36. Pappo AS, Armstrong GT, Liu W, et al. Melanoma as a subsequent neoplasm in adult survivors of childhood cancer: A report from the childhood cancer survivor study. Pediatr Blood Cancer 2013;60(3):461–6.
37. Hopkins ZH, Moreno C, Carlisle R, et al. Melanoma prognosis in the United States: Identifying barriers for improved care. J Am Acad Dermatol 2019;80(5):1256–62.
38. Vujic I, Gandini S, Stanganelli I, et al. A meta-analysis of melanoma risk in industrial workers. Melanoma Res 2018;1. https://doi.org/10.1097/CMR.0000000000000531.
39. Stanganelli I, De Felici MB, Mandel VD, et al. The association between pesticide use and cutaneous melanoma: a systematic review and meta-analysis. J Eur Acad Dermatol Venereol 2020;34(4):691–708.
40. US Preventive Services Task Force, Bibbins-Domingo K, Grossman DC, Curry SJ, et al. Screening for skin cancer: US Preventive Services Task Force Recommendation Statement. JAMA 2016;316:429.
41. Wolff T, Tai E, Miller T. Screening for skin cancer: an update of the evidence for the US Preventive Services Task Force. Ann Intern Med 2009;150:194.
42. Breitbart EW, Waldmann A, Nolte S, et al. Systematic skin cancer screening in Northern Germany. J Am Acad Dermatol 2012;66:201–9.
43. Waldmann A, Nolte S, Geller AC, et al. Frequency of excisions and yields of malignant skin tumors in a population-based screening intervention of 360,288 whole-body examinations. Arch Dermatol 2012;148:903–10.
44. Boniol M, Autier P, Gandini S. Melanoma mortality following skin cancer screening in Germany. BMJ Open 2015;5:e008158.

45. Katalinic A, Waldmann A, Weinstock MA, et al. Does skin cancer screening save lives?: an observational study comparing trends in melanoma mortality in regions with and without screening. Cancer 2012;118:5395–402.

46. Stang A, Jöckel KH. Does skin cancer screening save lives? A detailed analysis of mortality time trends in Schleswig-Holstein and Germany. Cancer 2016;122: 432–7.

47. Aitken JF, Elwood M, Baade PD, et al. Clinical whole-body skin examination reduces the incidence of thick melanomas. Int J Cancer 2010;126:450–8.

48. Ferris LK, Saul MI, Lin Y, et al. A large skin cancer screening quality initiative: description and first-year outcomes. JAMA Oncol 2017;3:1112–5.

49. Schneider JS, Moore DH 2nd, Mendelsohn ML. Screening program reduced melanoma mortality at the Lawrence Livermore National Laboratory, 1984 to 1996. J Am Acad Dermatol 2008;58:741–9.

50. Eide MJ, Asgari MM, Fletcher SW, et al. Effects on skills and practice from a web-based skin cancer course for primary care providers. J Am Board Fam Med 2013;26:648–57.

51. INFORMED: Melanoma and skin cancer early detection. Available at: http://www.skinsight.com/info/for_professionals/skin-cancer-detection-informed/skin-cancer-education. Accessed July 06, 2012.

52. Shaikh WR, Geller A, Alexander G, et al. Developing an interactive web-based learning program on skin cancer: the learning experiences of clinical educators. J Cancer Educ 2012;27:709–16.

53. Hoorens I, Vossaert K, Pil L, et al. Total-body examination vs lesion-directed skin cancer screening. JAMA Dermatol 2016;152:27–34.

54. Risica PM, Matthews NH, Dionne L, et al. Psychosocial consequences of skin cancer screening. Prev Med Rep 2018;10:310–6.

55. Winkler JK, Sies K, Fink C, et al. Melanoma recognition by a deep learning convolutional neural network-Performance in different melanoma subtypes and localisations. Eur J Cancer 2020;127:21–9.

56. Esteva A, Kuprel B, Novoa RA, et al. Dermatologist-level classification of skin cancer with deep neural networks. Nature 2017;542(7639):115–8.

Adjuvant Therapy of Melanoma

Ahmad A. Tarhini, MD, PhD[a,b,*]

KEYWORDS

- Adjuvant • Melanoma • Interferon • Ipilimumab • Pembrolizumab • Nivolumab
- Dabrafenib • Trametinib

KEY POINTS

- High-dose interferon-α regimen (HDI) approved in 1995 showed significant improvements in relapse-free survival (RFS) in 3 trials and overall survival (OS) in 2.
- Ipilimumab improved RFS compared with placebo and OS compared with placebo and HDI, albeit with a high toxicity and discontinuation rate.
- In cases in which adjuvant therapy with ipilimumab represents an option, the 3 mg/kg dose has an advantage over the approved dosage of 10 mg/kg.
- Nivolumab and pembrolizumab prolong RFS compared with ipilimumab or placebo, respectively and represent current first-line adjuvant standard of care.
- For BRAF mutated melanoma, dabrafenib plus trametinib prolong RFS compared with placebo and also represent current first-line standard of care for BRAF V600E/K mutated melanoma.

INTRODUCTION

Melanoma incidence continues to increase annually with 100,350 new cases and 6850 deaths estimated in the year 2020 in the United States.[1] High-risk melanoma can be defined as patients with deep primary tumors with or without surface ulceration (Stages IIB-C) or patients with regional nodal (stage III) or distant metastatic disease (stage IV) that can be rendered disease-free surgically, but are at a high risk for disease relapse and death from melanoma that increases with increasing stage. Systemic adjuvant therapy targeting residual micrometastatic disease which could be the source of future relapse can reduce the risk of relapse and improve survival as primarily tested in patients with stages III and IV. Among the adjuvant treatment modalities tested, immunotherapy with interferon-alfa (IFNα) and immune checkpoint inhibitors

[a] Department of Cutaneous Oncology, Moffitt Cancer Center and Research Institute, 10920 McKinley Drive, Tampa, FL 33612, USA; [b] Department of Immunology, Moffitt Cancer Center and Research Institute, 10902 USF Magnolia Drive, Tampa, FL 33612, USA
* Department of Cutaneous Oncology, Moffitt Cancer Center and Research Institute, 10920 McKinley Drive, Tampa, FL 33612, USA
E-mail address: Ahmad.Tarhini@Moffitt.org

Hematol Oncol Clin N Am 35 (2021) 73–84
https://doi.org/10.1016/j.hoc.2020.08.012
0889-8588/21/© 2020 Elsevier Inc. All rights reserved.

hemonc.theclinics.com

(ipilimumab, pembrolizumab, nivolumab) and targeted therapy with the BRAF-MEK inhibitors dabrafenib and trametinib have demonstrated significant improvements in the outcomes of patients with high-risk melanoma.

Melanoma risk of relapse and death can be estimated using key prognostic factors used by the American Joint Committee on Cancer (AJCC) staging system.[2] Stages I and II are defined as melanoma limited to the skin with no lymphatic or distant organ metastasis and constitutes stages I and II where the primary tumor thickness of invasion and the ulceration status define the stage groups (IA, IB, IIA, IIB, IIC). An increase in primary tumor thickness and the presence of ulceration correlate with a decrease in survival. An increase in mitotic rate of the primary tumor has been correlated with a decrease in melanoma patient survival but is not incorporated into the eighth edition of the AJCC staging system. Lymphatic nodal and/or in-transit metastases define stage III. Within stage III, the extent of nodal metastases whether microscopic or macroscopic and the number of involved lymph nodes indicate the stage groups where prognosis declines with increasing tumor burden (IIIA, IIIB, IIIC, IIID). Stage IV represents distant organ metastases. Within stage IV, distant cutaneous or nodal metastases (M1a) represent a better prognosis than lung (M1b), other visceral (M1c), or brain (M1d) metastases. Serum levels of lactate dehydrogenase (LDH) are associated with worse prognosis among patients with stage IV and appear to be a marker of tumor burden a marker of cancer metabolic activity and increased glucose uptake by tumor cells highly dependent on the anaerobic glycolytic pathway.[3]

Systemic adjuvant therapy is expected to benefit patients with melanoma with resected stages III and IV in which the risk of melanoma relapse ranges from approximately 40% to 90%.[4] Postoperative systemic adjuvant therapy targets residual regional or distant micrometastatic disease that could be the source of future melanoma relapse and has been shown to significantly improve relapse-free survival (RFS) and overall survival (OS) in this setting. By comparison, upfront or preoperative neoadjuvant systemic therapy presents an additional opportunity to improve the clinical outcome of patients with clinically detectable regionally advanced disease and has demonstrated promising results in early clinical trial testing.

ADJUVANT THERAPY WITH INTERFERON ALPHA

Interferon alpha-2 (IFNα) was studied extensively as systemic adjuvant therapy for high-risk melanoma with regimens that varied by dosage, route of administration, formulation, and duration of therapy.[5] The immune modulating effects of IFNα as studied in the neoadjuvant setting, include the induction of T-cell and dendritic cell infiltration into nodal metastases. It was shown to induce signal transducer and activator of transcription (STAT)1 upregulation while effecting STAT3 downregulation that may reverse T-cell signaling defects.[6] **Table 1** summarizes the key phase III adjuvant trials that impacted clinical practice.

Phase III Studies of Adjuvant High-Dose Interferon-α

Eastern Cooperative Oncology Group (ECOG) E1684 was the first trial to test high-dose IFNα (HDI) as adjuvant treatment for high-risk resected melanoma and led to regulatory approval by the US Food and Drug Administration in 1995.[7] This study randomized 287 patients to either HDI or observation. The HDI regimen began with an induction phase, which was given at 20 MU/m^2 of IFNα intravenously (IV) for 5 consecutive days a week for 4 weeks followed by a maintenance phase, that consisted of subcutaneous injections of 10 MU/m^2 3 times a week for 48 weeks. After a median follow-up of 6.9 years, the median RFS was 1.72 versus 0.98 years

Table 1
Randomized phase III trials of adjuvant interferon-α in resected melanoma divided by dose level

Trial	Number of Patients	Patient Population by Stage	Trial Arms	Regimen	Median Follow-up (y)	RFS	OS	Reference
High dose of IFNα								
NCCTG 83–7052	262	II-III (T2-4N0M0/TanyN + M0)	High-dose IFNα2a vs observation	IM 20 MU/m² 3 d/wk for 4 mo	6.1	NS	NS	Creagan, 1995
ECOG E1684	287	II-III (T4N0M0/TanyN + M0)	High-dose IFNα2b (HDI) vs observation	IV 20MU/m² 5 d/wk for 4 wk and then SC 10MU/m² 3 d/wk for 48 wk	6.9, 12.1	S	S (S at 6.9 y NS at 12.1 y)	Kirkwood et al,[7] 1996
ECOG E1690	642	II-III (T4N0M0/TanyN + M0)	HDI vs low dose vs observation	HDI IV 20 MU/m² 5 d/wk for 4 wk and then SC 10 MU/m² 3 d/wk for 48 wk IDI SC 3MU/m² 2 d/wk for 2 y	4.3, 6.6	S	NS	Kirkwood et al,[8] 2000
ECOG E1694	774	II-III (T4N0M0/TanyN + M0)	HDI vs GMK vaccine	IV 20MU/m² 5 d/wk for 4 wk and then SC 10 MU/m² 2 d/wk for 48 wk	1.3, 2.1	S	S	Kirkwood et al,[9] 2001
Italian Melanoma Intergroup	330	III (TanyN1-3M0)	Intensified IFNα2b (IHDI) every other mo vs HDI for 1 y	IHDI IV 20 MU/m² 5 d/wk for 4 wk every other mo for 4 cycles HDI IV 20 MU/m² 5 d/wk for 4 wk → then → SC 10 MU/m² 3 d/wk for 48 wk	5.0	NS	NS	Chiarion-Sileni, 2011
Medium dose of IFNα								
EORTC 18952	1388	II-III (T4N0M0/TanyN + M0)	IFNα2b for 1 y vs 2 y vs observation	IV 10 MU 5 d/wk for 4 wk and then (a) SC 10 MU 3 d/wk for 1 y OR (b) SC 5 MU 3 d/wk for 2 y	4.65	NS	NS	Eggermont, 2005

(continued on next page)

Table 1
(continued)

Trial	Number of Patients	Patient Population by Stage	Trial Arms	Regimen	Median Follow-up (y)	RFS	OS	Reference
EORTC 18991	1256	III (TanyN + M0)	PEG IFNα2b vs observation	SC 6 μg/kg/wk for 8 wk and then SC 3 μg/kg/wk for 5 y	3.8	S	NS	Eggermont et al,[12] 2008
Low dose of IFNα								
Austrian Melanoma Cooperative Group (AMCG)	311	II (T2-4N0M0)	IFNα2a vs observation	SC 3 MU 7 d/wk for 3 wk and then SC 3MU 3 d/wk for 1 y	3.4 (mean)	S	NS	Pehamberger, 1998
French Melanoma Cooperative Group (FCGM)	499	II (T2-4N0M0)	IFNα2a vs observation	SC 3 MU 3 d/wk for 3 y	>3	S	S	Grob, 1998
WHO-16	444	III (TanyN + M0)	IFNα2a vs observation	SC 3MU 3 d/wk for 3 y	7.3	NS	NS	Cascinelli, 1994
Scottish Melanoma Cooperative Group	96	II–III (T3-4N0M0/ TanyN + M0)	IFNα2a vs observation	SC 3 MU 3 d/wk for 6 mo	6.5	NS	NS	Cameron, 2001
EORTC 18871/ DKG-80	728	II–III (T3-4N0M0/ TanyN + M0)	IFNα2b vs IFNγ vs ISCADOR M® vs observation	IFNα2b: SC 1 MU every other day for 12 mo IFNγ: SC 0.2 mg every other day for 12 mo ISCADOR M	8.2	NS NS NS	NS NS NS	Kleeberg, 2004
UKCCCR/ AIM HIGH	674	II–III (T3-4N0M0/ TanyN + M0)	IFNα2a vs observation	IFN SC 3 MU 3 d/wk for 2 y	3.1	NS	NS	Hancock, 2004

DeCOG	840	III (T3anyN + M0)	IFNα2a for 18 mo (A) vs 3 y (B)	IFN SC 3MU 3 d/wk for 18 mo vs 3 y	4.3	NS	NS	Hauschild, 2010
DeCOG	441	III (TanyN + M0)	(A) IFNα2a (B) IFNα2a + dacarbazine (C) Observation	(A) IFN SC 3MU 3 d/wk for 24 mo (B) IFN SC 3MU 3 d/wk for 24 mo + DTIC 850 mg/m^2 every 4–8 wk for 24 mo	3.9	S NS	S NS	Garbe, 2008

Abbreviations: HDI, high-dose IFN; IFN, interferon; IV, intravenous; LDI, low-dose IFN; MU, million units; NS, nonsignificant; OS, overall survival; RFS, relapse-free survival; S, statistically significant improvement reported; SC, subcutaneous.

(P = .0023) with a hazard ratio (HR) of 0.61 (P = .0013), and the median OS was 3.82 versus 2.78 years (P = .0237), HR = 0.67 (P = .01). Patients with lymph node involvement (N1 disease) appeared to primarily derive the survival benefit seen in this study. However, HDI was associated with significant toxicity, in which the incidence of grade 3 and 4 adverse events was 67% and 9% respectively, including 2 hepatotoxic deaths. E1690 (N = 642) tested HDI and a low dose of IFNα (LDI; 3 MU subcutaneously [SC] thrice weekly for 2 years) and failed to demonstrate OS benefit with either regimen compared with observation.[8] Unlike E1684, this study did not require elective lymph node dissection and a retrospective analysis suggested that 38 patients with regional nodal relapse on observation received HDI as adjuvant therapy that may have affected the survival analysis. On the other hand, after a median follow-up of 4.3 years, significant improvement in RFS was seen with HDI. E1694 (N = 880) compared adjuvant therapy with a ganglioside vaccine (GMK) with HDI. The investigation of GMK in this setting was based on prior studies that had shown evidence of immunogenicity and suggested clinical activity. After a 2.1 year median follow-up, HDI was superior in OS (HR = 0.72) and RFS (HR = 0.67) as compared with the vaccine.[9] The 2 observation-controlled trials (E1684 and E1690) were pooled in an analysis that was updated through April 2001. After a median follow-up of 12.6 years for E1684 and 6.6 years for E1690, the analysis concluded that there was no significant benefit in OS benefit for HDI compared with observation. RFS benefits in favor of HDI continued to be seen with this long term follow-up.[10] This was consistent with the findings from the larger of the 2 trials (E1690) that did not show an OS improvement with HDI. E1697 targeted intermediate risk melanoma patients with either node negative disease (T2bN0, T3a-bN0, T4a-bN0) or microscopic nodal disease (N1a-N2a).[11] Patients (N = 1150) who were randomized to either observation or 4 weeks of HDI IV at 20 MU/m^2 per day, 5 days per week. HDI failed to demonstrate any RFS or OS benefits in this trial.

Adjuvant Therapy with Pegylated Interferon-α

Pegylated IFNα (peg-IFN) was developed to have sustained absorption and a longer half-life. EORTC 18991 tested peg-IFN in resected stage III melanoma as compared with observation. The peg-IFN adjuvant regimen was given SC and consisted of an induction phase (6 μg/kg a week for 8 weeks) and a maintenance phase (3 μg/kg a week for up to 5 years). At a median follow-up of 7.6 years, there was a modest improvement in RFS in favor of peg-IFN (HR = 0.87), but no OS benefits. The regimen was also toxic having a 37% toxicity attrition rate. A subgroup analysis suggested that patients with microscopic nodal metastasis and among this group, patients with an ulcerated primary, may have benefited the most from adjuvant peg-IFN.[12]

Meta-Analyses of Randomized Controlled Trials Testing Adjuvant Interferon-α

Four meta-analyses of randomized controlled trials (RCTs) of adjuvant IFNα in melanoma were conducted.[13–15] The largest and more recent meta-analysis was the Cochrane Analysis of Adjuvant Melanoma Trials.[15] This meta-analysis included 17 RCTs and a total of 10,499 patients and concluded modest RFS (HR 0.83; 95% confidence interval [CI] 0.78–0.87) and OS (HR 0.91; 95% CI 0.85–0.97) benefits with adjuvant IFNα.

ADJUVANT BIOCHEMOTHERAPY

The S0008 study was conducted by the South West Oncology Group and compared adjuvant therapy with the E1684 HDI regimen with a 9-week biochemotherapy (BCT) regimen consisting of 3 cycles of cisplatin, vinblastine, and dacarbazine, and low doses of interleukin (IL)-2 and IFNα.[16] At a median follow-up of 7.2 years, there was an improvement in RFS in favor of BCT (median RFS of 4.0 vs 1.9 years; HR 0.75, 95% CI 0.58–0.97); however, there was no difference in the OS rates. BCT had a higher toxicity rate with grade 3 to 4 adverse event rates of 76% and 64%.

ADJUVANT IMMUNOTHERAPY WITH VACCINES

Vaccines tested as adjuvant therapy in melanoma included whole cells (cell lysates), peptide vaccines, and ganglioside antigen vaccines, but have generally failed to demonstrate significant benefits. One approach investigated an allogeneic whole-cell vaccine (Canvaxin) plus bacillus Calmette-Guerin (BCG) as compared with BCG in resected stage III and IV melanoma.[17] The DERMA adjuvant trial tested the Melanoma antigen A (MAGE)-A3 Cancer/Testis antigen protein vaccine given with the AS15 immunostimulant in patients with stage IIIB or IIIC MAGE-A3-positive cutaneous melanoma.[18]

ADJUVANT THERAPY WITH BEVACIZUMAB

Vascular endothelial growth factor inhibition with bevacizumab was investigated in the phase III AVAST-M trial as compared with observation in patients with resected AJCC stages II and III melanoma.[19] Disease-free interval was significantly, although modestly improved with favor of bevacizumab (HR 0.83; 95% CI 0.70–0.98; $P = .03$). However, there were no significant differences in OS or distant metastasis-free survival after a median follow-up of 25 months.

ADJUVANT THERAPY WITH IPILIMUMAB

CTLA-4 blockade with ipilimumab demonstrated significant clinical benefits leading to regulatory approval for metastatic melanoma at the dose of 3 mg/kg and resected stage III melanoma at 10 mg/kg. The pivotal MDX10 to 20 trial in metastatic melanoma tested ipilimumab at 3 mg/kg every 3 weeks for 4 doses as compared with the combination of ipilimumab and a peptide vaccine, and vaccine-placebo.[20] Ipilimumab significantly improved survival compared with the vaccine leading to regulatory approval at this dose level. Another study evaluating ipilimumab at 10 mg/kg combined with dacarbazine compared with dacarbazine was also positive (CA 184–024).[21]

EORTC 18071 was a placebo-controlled adjuvant trial that tested ipilimumab at 10 mg/kg every 3 weeks for 4 doses then every 3 months for up to 3 years in patients with stage IIIA (N2a), IIIB, and IIIC melanoma (except in-transit disease).[22] At a median follow-up of 2.7 years, median RFS was 26.1 months versus 17.1 months (HR 0.75; 95% CI 0.64–0.90; $P = .0013$). Adjuvant ipilimumab at 10 mg/kg was associated with significant toxicity, including 5 events of death as a result of immune related adverse events. A later update with a median follow-up of 5.3 years, confirmed the RFS benefits and reported significant OS improvement. The 5-year OS rate was 65.4% versus 54.4% (HR 0.72; 95% CI 0.58–0.88; $P = .001$).[23] These benefits were further confirmed in a more recent update with a median follow-up of 6.9 years.

NORTH AMERICAN INTERGROUP E1609

E1609 is the largest adjuvant trial in melanoma with participation from 1673 patients.[24] Following the regulatory approval of ipilimumab at 3 mg/kg (ipi3) for metastatic unresectable melanoma and the later approval of adjuvant ipilimumab at 10 mg/kg (ipi10), the relative safety and efficacy of ipilimumab at the 2 dose levels became important to evaluate compared with high-dose interferon-alfa (HDI), a standard adjuvant treatment for high-risk melanoma available since 1996. E1609 compared ipilimumab at 3 and 10 mg/kg with HDI in patients with resected stages IIIB, IIIC (including resected in-transit disease), M1a, M1b with participation from 850 sites across the United States and Canada. Patients were randomly assigned 1:1:1 between May 2011 and August 2014 to receive ipi3 (n = 523), HDI (n = 636), or ipi10 (n = 511). Ipilimumab was given every 3 weeks for 4 doses as induction therapy, followed by every 12 weeks for up to 4 additional doses as maintenance. At a median follow-up of 57.4 months, ipi3 was significantly superior to HDI in the primary endpoint of OS (HR 0.78%; 95.6% repeated CI 0.61–0.99; P = .044), whereas for RFS, HR was 0.85 (99.4% CI 0.66–1.09; P = .065). Median OS at 5 years was 72% versus 67% and median RFS was 4.5 versus 2.5 years. The comparison of ipi10 versus HDI was not significant. Furthermore, ipi10 was significantly more toxic than ipi3.

ADJUVANT THERAPY WITH ANTI-PD-1 ANTIBODIES

CheckMate-238 was a phase III study that tested adjuvant nivolumab (3 mg/kg every 2 weeks) versus ipilimumab (10 mg/kg every 3 weeks for 4 doses then every 12 weeks) for up to 1 year in patients with stage IIIB, IIIC, or IV melanoma.[25] The study met its primary endpoint of RFS at a minimum follow-up of 18 months. At 12 months, RFS was 70.5% with and 60.8% with ipilimumab (HR 0.65; 97.56% CI 0.51–0.83; P<.001). The rate of treatment-related grade 3 to 4 adverse events was 14.4% in the nivolumab group and the toxicity attrition rate was 9.7%.

KEYNOTE-054 tested adjuvant therapy with pembrolizumab versus placebo in patients with resected stage III melanoma having stage IIIA (N1a; at least 1 micrometastasis >1 mm), stage IIIB and IIIC (no in-transit metastases).[26] The primary endpoints included RFS in the overall population and in the PD-L1 positive subgroup. Both endpoints were met after a median follow-up of 15 months. The 1-year RFS rate was 75.4% versus 61.0% (HR 0.57; 98.4% CI 0.43–0.74; P<.001). In PD-L1–positive, 1-year RFS was 77.1% versus 62.6% (HR 0.54, 95% CI 0.42–0.69; P<.001). The rate of grades 3 to 5 treatment-related adverse events was 14.7% in the pembrolizumab group with 1 treatment-related death due to myositis. The toxicity attrition rate was 13.0%.

Ongoing studies testing anti-PD1 antibodies include S1404 that is investigating pembrolizumab versus the choice of either HDI or ipilimumab at 10 mg/kg in melanoma patients with resected stage IIIA(N2), IIIB, IIIC, and IV. This study completed accrual in August 2017.

CheckMate-915 is a randomized phase III study evaluating adjuvant therapy with nivolumab (240 mg every 2 weeks) plus ipilimumab (1 mg/kg every 6 weeks) versus nivolumab (480 mg every 4 weeks) for 1 year in patients with resected AJCC 8th edition stage IIIB, IIIC, IIID, and IV melanoma. The study has 2 co-primary endpoints that include RFS in the intent-to-treat population and RFS in the PD-L1 negative (<1%) patient population. A press release by Bristol Myers Squibb on November 20, 2019 reported that there was no statistically significant benefit in the co-primary endpoint of RFS in PD-L1 negative patients. The study continues double-blinded to assess the other co-primary endpoint.

ADJUVANT TARGETED THERAPY WITH DABRAFENIB AND TRAMETINIB

COMBI-AD was a phase III study that tested adjuvant therapy with dabrafenib and trametinib for 1 year as compared with placebo in patients with resected stage IIIA (lymph node metastasis of >1 mm), IIIB ,or IIIC (according to AJCC seventh edition) and BRAF V600E/K mutation-positive melanoma.[27] The primary endpoint was RFS and this was significantly improved. After a median follow-up of 44 months for dabrafenib plus trametinib, the 3-year and 4-year RFS rates were 59% and 54% in the treatment group versus 40% and 38% in the placebo group, respectively (HR 0.49; 95% CI 0.40–0.59). Using a Weibull mixture cure-rate model for RFS, the estimated cure rate was 54% with dabrafenib plus trametinib compared with 37% with placebo. With dabrafenib plus trametinib, adverse events led to permanent discontinuation of a trial drug in 26%, dose reduction in 38%, and dose interruption in 66%.

BRIM-8 tested adjuvant vemurafenib versus placebo in patients with stages IIC-IIIA-IIIB (cohort 1) melanoma or stage IIIC (cohort 2) BRAF V600 mutation-positive melanoma.[28] The primary endpoint was disease-free survival (DFS) as tested separately in each cohort following a hierarchical analytical approach with cohort 2 prespecified before cohort 1. Overall, 184 patients were enrolled in cohort 2 and 314 patients in cohort 1. After a median study follow-up of 33.5 months, in patients with stage IIIC (cohort 2), median DFS was 23.1 months with vemurafenib versus 15.4 months with placebo (HR 0.80; 95% CI 0.54–1.18; P = .26). In patients with stage IIC-IIIA-IIIB, median DFS was not reached in the vemurafenib arm versus 36.9 months in the placebo arm (HR 0.54; 95% CI 0.37–0.78; P = .0010). This result in cohort 1 was not considered significant owing to the prespecified hierarchical prerequisite.

ADJUVANT RADIATION THERAPY

Studies of adjuvant radiation therapy for highest risk melanoma have demonstrated improvements in reducing the risk of local relapse, but have failed to show significant benefits in RFS or OS.[29–32] A study retrospectively reviewed 160 patients with regionally advanced melanoma who received adjuvant radiotherapy (30 Gy in 6-Gy fractions given twice per week) following surgical resection. The study suggested improvements in locoregional disease control.[29] Similar results were suggested by another retrospective study that evaluated regional recurrence rate for postoperative adjuvant radiotherapy compared with surgery alone.[33] A later retrospective study in patients with regionally advanced melanoma to the neck and/or parotid, reported benefits in locoregional disease control.[31] A later randomized trial evaluated adjuvant radiotherapy (48 Gy in 20 fractions) compared with postoperative observation among 217 patients with regional lymph node metastases and high-risk features for recurrence, including extranodal tumor extension, the number of lymph nodes involved and the size of involved lymph nodes.[30] After a median follow-up of 40 months, the risk of lymph-node field relapse was improved (HR 0.56; 95% CI 0.32–0.98; P = .041); however, there were no significant differences in RFS or OS.

DISCUSSION

The goal of systemic adjuvant therapy for resected cutaneous melanoma that is at high risk for disease relapse and death is targeting residual micrometastatic disease that could be the source of future relapse. IFNα was extensively studied in regimens that varied by dosage, route of administration, formulation, and duration of therapy. The high-dose regimen (HDI) showed significant improvements in RFS in 3 RCTs (E1684, E1690, E1694) and OS in 2. Peg-IFN modestly reduced the risk of relapse with no impact on OS as studied in the EORTC 18991 trial. More recently (EORTC 18071), ipilimumab at the high dose of 10 mg/kg (ipi10) was shown to significantly improve RFS and OS but at a significant toxicity cost (EORTC 18071). North American Intergroup E1609 tested ipilimumab at 3 mg/kg (ipi3) or ipi10 versus HDI and demonstrated significant OS benefits with ipi3 compared with HDI and less toxicity compared with ipi10. E1609 was unique in having 2 co-primary endpoints, OS and RFS. For the first time in melanoma adjuvant therapy, this study has demonstrated a significant improvement in OS against an active control regimen. The data supported the use of ipi3 over HDI based on improved survival and similar RFS, and comparable toxicity and that in cases in which adjuvant therapy with ipilimumab represents an option, ipi3 had an advantage over the approved dosage of ipi10. More recently, the standard of care has changed in favor of the anti-PD1 antibodies nivolumab (CheckMate-238; vs ipi10) and pembrolizumab (KEYNOTE-054; vs placebo) based on significant RFS benefits. Similarly, RFS was significantly improved with dabrafenib plus trametinib in patients with BRAF mutated melanoma (COMBI-AD; vs placebo). The clinical benefits were similar when comparing the studies that tested anti-PD1 or dabrafenib and trametinib with no clear advantage for either in patients with BRAF mutated melanoma. The choice of therapy may depend on preferences related to the route of administration and on the respective toxicity profiles. A recent systematic literature review using Bayesian network meta-analysis investigated RFS distant metastasis free survival and OS in adjuvant trials that tested dabrafenib plus trametinib, nivolumab, pembrolizumab, ipilimumab, vemurafenib, chemotherapy, and IFNα.[34] The study concluded that efficacy was comparable between targeted therapy (dabrafenib plus trametinib) and anti-PD1 checkpoint inhibitors. In drug development, the neoadjuvant approach provides the ability to evaluate clinical and radiologic tumor responses along with pathologic responses and potentially improve the clinical outcome for regionally advanced operable melanoma. Neoadjuvant therapy using immune checkpoint inhibitors and BRAF-MEK inhibitors has demonstrated promising data in early trials that have started to impact the standard of care and phase III testing is currently underway.

SUMMARY

For resected high-risk melanoma, significant benefits have been demonstrated in RCTs testing adjuvant therapy with IFNα (HDI and peg-IFN), ipilimumab, nivolumab, pembrolizumab and dabrafenib plus trametinib (for BRAF V600E/K mutated melanoma) leading to regulatory approvals. E1609 is the largest adjuvant trial in melanoma and was the first to demonstrate significant improvement in OS with ipi3 compared with an active control. The current first-line adjuvant standard of care consists of anti-PD1 immunotherapy with pembrolizumab and nivolumab as well as targeted therapy with dabrafenib plus trametinib for BRAF V600E/K mutated melanoma. In patients in whom adjuvant ipilimumab represents an option, ipi3 has an advantage over the approved dosage of ipi10.

DISCLOSURE

A.A. Tarhini reported consulting fees from Bristol Myers Squibb, Novartis, Genentech-Roche, Partner Therapeutics. Contracted research funding from Oncosec, Clinigen (outside the submitted work).

REFERENCES

1. Siegel RL, Miller KD, Jemal A. Cancer statistics, 2020. CA Cancer J Clin 2020; 70(1):7–30.

2. Gershenwald JE, Scolyer RA, Hess KR, et al. Melanoma staging: evidence-based changes in the American Joint Committee on Cancer eighth edition cancer staging manual. CA Cancer J Clin 2017;67(6):472–92.

3. Feron O. Pyruvate into lactate and back: from the Warburg effect to symbiotic energy fuel exchange in cancer cells. Radiother Oncol 2009;92(3):329–33.

4. Romano E, Scordo M, Dusza SW, et al. Site and timing of first relapse in stage III melanoma patients: implications for follow-up guidelines. J Clin Oncol 2010; 28(18):3042–7.

5. Hodi FS, Lee S, McDermott DF, et al. Ipilimumab plus sargramostim vs ipilimumab alone for treatment of metastatic melanoma: a randomized clinical trial. JAMA 2014;312(17):1744–53.

6. Kirkwood JM, Moschos S, Wang W. Strategies for the development of more effective adjuvant therapy of melanoma: current and future explorations of antibodies, cytokines, vaccines, and combinations. Clin Cancer Res 2006;12(7 Pt 2): 2331s–6s.

7. Kirkwood JM, Strawderman MH, Ernstoff MS, et al. Interferon alfa-2b adjuvant therapy of high-risk resected cutaneous melanoma: the Eastern Cooperative Oncology Group Trial EST 1684. J Clin Oncol 1996;14(1):7–17.

8. Kirkwood JM, Ibrahim JG, Sondak VK, et al. High- and low-dose interferon alfa-2b in high-risk melanoma: first analysis of intergroup trial E1690/S9111/C9190. J Clin Oncol 2000;18(12):2444–58.

9. Kirkwood JM, Ibrahim JG, Sosman JA, et al. High-dose interferon alfa-2b significantly prolongs relapse-free and overall survival compared with the GM2-KLH/QS-21 vaccine in patients with resected stage IIB-III melanoma: results of intergroup trial E1694/S9512/C509801. J Clin Oncol 2001;19(9):2370–80.

10. Kirkwood JM, Manola J, Ibrahim J, et al. A pooled analysis of eastern cooperative oncology group and intergroup trials of adjuvant high-dose interferon for melanoma. Clin Cancer Res 2004;10(5):1670–7.

11. Agarwala SS, Lee SJ, Yip W, et al. Phase III randomized study of 4 weeks of high-dose interferon-alpha-2b in stage T2bNO, T3a-bNO, T4a-bNO, and T1-4N1a-2a (microscopic) melanoma: a trial of the Eastern Cooperative Oncology Group-American College of Radiology Imaging Network Cancer Research Group (E1697). J Clin Oncol 2017;35(8):885–92.

12. Eggermont AM, Suciu S, Santinami M, et al. Adjuvant therapy with pegylated interferon alfa-2b versus observation alone in resected stage III melanoma: final results of EORTC 18991, a randomised phase III trial. Lancet 2008;372(9633): 117–26.

13. Wheatley K, Ives N, Hancock B, et al. Does adjuvant interferon-alpha for high-risk melanoma provide a worthwhile benefit? A meta-analysis of the randomised trials. Cancer Treat Rev 2003;29(4):241–52.

14. Wheatley K, Ives N, Eggermont A, et al. Interferon-α as adjuvant therapy for melanoma: An individual patient data meta-analysis of randomised trials. Journal of Clinical Oncology 2007;25(18suppl):8526-8526.

15. Mocellin S, Lens MB, Pasquali S, et al. Interferon alpha for the adjuvant treatment of cutaneous melanoma. Cochrane Database Syst Rev 2013;6:CD008955.

16. Flaherty LE, Othus M, Atkins MB, et al. Southwest Oncology Group S0008: a phase III trial of high-dose interferon Alfa-2b versus cisplatin, vinblastine, and dacarbazine, plus interleukin-2 and interferon in patients with high-risk melanoma–an intergroup study of cancer and leukemia Group B, Children's Oncology Group, Eastern Cooperative Oncology Group, and Southwest Oncology Group. J Clin Oncol 2014;32(33):3771–8.

17. Faries MB, Mozzillo N, Kashani-Sabet M, et al. Long-term survival after complete surgical resection and adjuvant immunotherapy for distant melanoma metastases. Ann Surg Oncol 2017;24(13):3991–4000.

18. Dreno B, Thompson JF, Smithers BM, et al. MAGE-A3 immunotherapeutic as adjuvant therapy for patients with resected, MAGE-A3-positive, stage III melanoma (DERMA): a double-blind, randomised, placebo-controlled, phase 3 trial. Lancet Oncol 2018;19(7):916–29.
19. Corrie PG, Marshall A, Dunn JA, et al. Adjuvant bevacizumab in patients with melanoma at high risk of recurrence (AVAST-M): preplanned interim results from a multicentre, open-label, randomised controlled phase 3 study. Lancet Oncol 2014;15(6):620–30.
20. Hodi FS, O'Day SJ, McDermott DF, et al. Improved survival with ipilimumab in patients with metastatic melanoma. N Engl J Med 2010;363(8):711–23.
21. Robert C, Thomas L, Bondarenko I, et al. Ipilimumab plus dacarbazine for previously untreated metastatic melanoma. N Engl J Med 2011;364(26):2517–26.
22. Eggermont AM, Chiarion-Sileni V, Grob JJ, et al. Adjuvant ipilimumab versus placebo after complete resection of high-risk stage III melanoma (EORTC 18071): a randomised, double-blind, phase 3 trial. Lancet Oncol 2015;16(5):522–30.
23. Eggermont AM, Chiarion-Sileni V, Grob JJ, et al. Prolonged survival in stage III melanoma with ipilimumab adjuvant therapy. N Engl J Med 2016;375(19): 1845–55.
24. Tarhini AA, Lee SJ, Hodi FS, et al. Phase III study of adjuvant ipilimumab (3 or 10 mg/kg) versus high-dose interferon alfa-2b for resected high-risk melanoma: North American Intergroup E1609. J Clin Oncol 2020;38(6):567–75.
25. Weber J, Mandala M, Del Vecchio M, et al. Adjuvant nivolumab versus ipilimumab in resected stage III or IV melanoma. N Engl J Med 2017;377(19):1824–35.
26. Eggermont AMM, Blank CU, Mandala M, et al. Adjuvant pembrolizumab versus placebo in resected stage III melanoma. N Engl J Med 2018;378(19):1789–801.
27. Hauschild A, Dummer R, Schadendorf D, et al. Longer follow-up confirms relapse-free survival benefit with adjuvant dabrafenib plus trametinib in patients with resected BRAF V600-mutant stage III melanoma. J Clin Oncol 2018;36(35): 3441–9.
28. Maio M, Lewis K, Demidov L, et al. Adjuvant vemurafenib in resected, BRAF(V600) mutation-positive melanoma (BRIM8): a randomised, double-blind, placebo-controlled, multicentre, phase 3 trial. Lancet Oncol 2018;19(4):510–20.
29. Ballo MT, Ang KK. Radiation therapy for malignant melanoma. Surg Clin North Am 2003;83(2):323–42.
30. Burmeister BH, Henderson MA, Ainslie J, et al. Adjuvant radiotherapy versus observation alone for patients at risk of lymph-node field relapse after therapeutic lymphadenectomy for melanoma: a randomised trial. Lancet Oncol 2012;13(6): 589–97.
31. Strojan P, Jancar B, Cemazar M, et al. Melanoma metastases to the neck nodes: role of adjuvant irradiation. Int J Radiat Oncol Biol Phys 2010;77(4):1039–45.
32. Agrawal S, Kane JM 3rd, Guadagnolo BA, et al. The benefits of adjuvant radiation therapy after therapeutic lymphadenectomy for clinically advanced, high-risk, lymph node-metastatic melanoma. Cancer 2009;115(24):5836–44.
33. Khan N, Khan MK, Almasan A, et al. The evolving role of radiation therapy in the management of malignant melanoma. Int J Radiat Oncol Biol Phys 2011;80(3): 645–54.
34. Sharma R, Koruth R, Kanters S, et al. Comparative efficacy and safety of dabrafenib in combination with trametinib versus competing adjuvant therapies for high-risk melanoma. J Comp Eff Res 2019;8(16):1349–63.

Extracutaneous Melanoma

Richard Carvajal, MD[a],*, Rohan Maniar, MD[b]

KEYWORDS

- Mucosal melanoma • Anorectal melanoma • Vulvovaginal melanoma
- Uveal melanoma • Ocular melanoma • Systemic therapy

KEY POINTS

- Extracutaneous melanoma includes mucosal and uveal melanoma, which have distinct molecular features compared with cutaneous melanoma.
- Both diseases are characterized high rates of distant metastasis despite local control.
- Current treatments, including immune checkpoint blockade and targeted therapies, have not yielded the same benefits as are seen in cutaneous melanoma.
- Uveal melanoma has distinct mutations with GNAQ/GNA11 and BRCA1-associated protein 1, with targeted therapies currently under investigation.

INTRODUCTION

Melanoma is a clinically and molecularly diverse disease that encompasses a wide range of subtypes and presentation features. It has only been in recent years that understanding of the molecular and immunologic framework for this disease has led to meaningful treatment options. Within melanoma is a constellation of rare subtypes and presentations, including melanoma with brain metastases and leptomeningeal disease, acral melanoma, pediatric melanoma, and melanoma of unknown primary, as well as uncommon sites of presentation such as extracutaneous melanoma (ECMs). Therefore, melanoma research has had to remain at the forefront of development with inclusion of special populations that would otherwise be excluded from most therapeutic clinical trials.

ECMs share an aggressive natural history and higher mortalities owing, in part, to the rarity of these diseases and the lack of robust clinical trial data. Many of the management recommendations are based on consensus opinion or extrapolated from the experiences with nonacral cutaneous melanoma (NACM), resulting in poorer

[a] Experimental Therapeutics & Melanoma Service, Division of Hematology/Oncology, Columbia University Irving Medical Center, Milstein Hospital Building, 177 Fort Washington Avenue, 6GN-435, New York, NY 10032, USA; [b] Division of Hematology/Oncology, Columbia University Irving Medical Center, Milstein Hospital Building, 177 Fort Washington Avenue, 6GN-435, New York, NY 10032, USA
* Corresponding author.
E-mail address: rdc2150@cumc.columbia.edu

Hematol Oncol Clin N Am 35 (2021) 85–98
https://doi.org/10.1016/j.hoc.2020.09.004
0889-8588/21/© 2020 Elsevier Inc. All rights reserved.

outcomes. Despite these sobering characteristics, emerging treatments have begun to provide improved clinical benefits and reshape the trajectory of the disease course.

This article discusses ECMs. It reviews the epidemiology, natural history, clinical and molecular features, and treatment options for mucosal and uveal melanoma. It focuses on the genetic and immunologic characteristics that rationalize the use of systemic therapies both in the adjuvant and advanced disease settings. In addition, it reviews emerging research and therapeutic options that have expanded the armamentarium for treatment.

MUCOSAL MELANOMA
Epidemiology and Clinical Features

Mucosal melanoma (MM) is extremely rare, representing approximately 0.03% of all new cancer diagnoses and 1.4% of all melanomas in the United States.[1] Although the incidence of NACM has continued to increase over the last 4 decades, MM has remained relatively stable.[2] MM arises from melanocytes on glabrous surfaces, typically in the respiratory, gastrointestinal (GI), and urogenital tracts. The most common sites of occurrence include the head and neck (55.4%), anorectal region (23.8%), and vulvovaginal region (18.0%). Rare sites of disease include the urinary tract, upper and lower GI tract (eg, esophagus and duodenum), and the gallbladder (**Table 1**).

MM has a higher incidence rate in women (2.8 vs 1.5 cases per 1 million) and tends to occur in older patients with a median age of 70 years at the time of diagnosis.[1,2] An important feature of MM is the varied incidence rates among different ethnic groups. Although the disease remains rare in white populations, rates of up to 39.6% of all melanoma cases arise in Asian populations.[3] Black South African and Hispanic populations have higher rates of MM, comprising 10% and 4%, respectively, of all melanoma cases[4] (**Table 2**).

Although NACM is frequently characterized by progression of precursor melanocytic nevi, mucosal melanocytic nevi do not seem to act as precursors. Multifocal disease is often seen at the time of presentation[5] and, advanced disease is found in approximately half of patients at the time of diagnosis. Amelanotic melanoma can occur in approximately 40% of patients, with clinical disease resembling other malignancies delaying diagnosis.[6]

Pathogenesis and Natural History

The pathogenesis of MM remains incompletely elucidated, although recent discoveries have found aberrant intracellular signaling pathways (discussed later).

Table 1		
Presenting signs and symptoms of mucosal melanoma by anatomic site		
Head and Neck (eg, Oral Cavity or Sinonasal Cavity)	**Anorectal**	**Vulvovaginal**
• Direct observation of a hyperpigmented lesion	• Rectal bleeding	• Mass
• Nasal obstruction	• Anorectal mass	• Pain
• Epistaxis	• Tenesmus	• Bleeding
• Tooth mobility	• Suspicion of hemorrhoids	• Pruritus
• Oral bleeding	• Incontinence	• Discharge
	• Inguinal mass	• Dyspareunia
	• Pruritus	
	• Change in bowel habits	
	• Weight loss	

Table 2 Distribution of mucosal melanoma by ethnic background		
Mucosal Melanoma Anatomic Distribution	Lian et al,[61] 2017	Patrick et al,[62] 2007
Head and neck (%)	38.0	55.4
Anorectal (%)	26.5	23.8
Vulvovaginal (%)	22.5	18.0
Other (%)	13.0	2.8

Data from Lian, B., et al., The natural history and patterns of metastases from mucosal melanoma: an analysis of 706 prospectively followed patients. Ann Oncol, 2017. 28(4): p. 868-873 And Patrick, R.J., N.A. Fenske, and J.L. Messina, Primary mucosal melanoma. J Am Acad Dermatol, 2007. 56(5): p. 828-34.

Historically, patients with MM have had substantially poorer outcomes compared with patients with NACM, with a 5-year survival of 80.8% versus 25.0% in patients with NACM.[2,7] This finding is attributable to the higher rates of advanced disease at the time of diagnosis, as shown by regional lymph node involvement (21% head and neck, 61% anorectal, and 23% vulvovaginal) compared with cutaneous disease (9%).[2] Five-year survival differed among patients with MM based on anatomic distribution as well. Head and neck, anorectal, and vulvovaginal distributions were associated with 5-year survival of 31.7%, 19.8%, and 11.4%, respectively.

Molecular Features and Immune Biology

Unlike NACM, which is notable for a high burden of somatic mutations, MM tends to have significantly fewer mutations despite being a molecularly heterogeneous disease. Whole-genome sequencing (WGS) of NACM typically carries 30,000 somatic single nucleotide variants (SNVs) per genome compared with only 8000 SNVs per genome in MM with an overall burden of approximately 2.7 mutations per megabase.[8–10] A meta-analysis of MM somatic mutations using targeted sequencing or whole-exome sequencing/WGS of tumor tissue highlighted the contrasting mutational landscape of MM compared with NACM.[11]

As noted in **Fig. 1**, mutations within the mitogen-associated protein kinase (MAPK) pathway (eg, BRAF, NRAS, NF1) occur at lower rates in MM compared with the cutaneous melanoma, as shown by The Cancer Genome Atlas (TCGA) data. Mucosal disease found in the lower region (eg, lower GI tract, anorectal and genital areas) shows a higher mutational burden of SF3B1 compared with disease in the upper region (eg, oral cavity, nasal cavity, and upper GI tract). SF3B1 is a spliceosomal protein that plays a role in RNA splicing, which promotes maturation of RNA transcripts. Mutations in SF3B1 have been identified in other conditions such as myelodysplastic syndrome (MDS), chronic lymphocytic leukemia, uveal melanoma, and breast cancer.

KIT is a transmembrane receptor tyrosine kinase that regulates normal cell growth and proliferation for melanocytes via downstream pathways of MAPK, AKT, and JAK/STAT. Aberrant expression with gain-of-function activity has been observed in numerous malignancies, including breast cancer, small cell lung cancer, GIST, and small cell lung cancer. As many as 39% of patients with MM harbor KIT alterations.[12] Both mammalian target of rapamycin (mTOR) pathway (PI3K-AKT-mTOR) and GNAQ or GNA11 mutations are seen in up to 14% and 10% of MM tumors, respectively, and

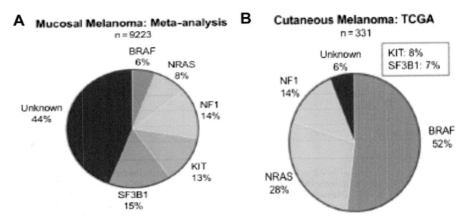

Fig. 1. Mutational landscape of MM (*A*) and cutaneous melanoma (*B*). (*From* Nassarab, K.W. and Tan, A.C. The mutational landscape of mucosal melanoma. Seminars in Cancer Biology 2020;60: 139-148.)

are associated with poor outcomes compared with tumors without those mutations.[13,14] An analysis of 213 tumor samples found amplification of CDK4 and CCND1 in 47% and 27.7%, respectively, and deletion of P16^{INK4a} in 57.7%.[15] The mutational landscape for MM has continued to evolve with deep sequencing and larger sample cohorts.

The unique environment from which MM arises has strong implications for the immunologic phenotype. Immunohistochemistry analysis of MM tumors found programmed death-ligand 1 (PD-L1) expression in 44% of samples and broad presence of tumor-infiltrating lymphocytes (TILs).[16]

THERAPEUTIC OPTIONS
Surgical Management

The primary treatment of MM is wide local excision, regardless of primary site, for localized and locally advanced disease. For head and neck MM (HNMM), surgical approaches using endoscopic techniques can help with decreasing the complications and morbidity associated with resection.[17] For anorectal disease, sphincter-sparing surgery is the preferred approach to reduce morbidity; however, abdominoperineal resection may provide better local control compared with local excision.[18] For vulvovaginal disease, wide local excision is preferred rather than pelvic exenteration because of high recurrence of distant disease despite aggressive surgical approaches. Despite local control, more than 50% of patients go on to develop distant metastasis.

Radiation Therapy

Adjuvant and definitive radiation therapy (RT) may be used in patients with locally advanced disease or patients for whom resection is not feasible. Adjuvant RT can provide additional benefit for local control but does not seem to influence overall survival (OS). RT has been used for HNMM in both the adjuvant and definitive settings when surgery is not feasible. In addition, the incorporation of newer techniques, including use of intensity-modulated RT, neutrons, carbon-ion therapy, and proton therapy, has helped to decrease radiation-induced toxicities and enhance therapeutic efficacy.

However, these advances have not yielded meaningful improvements on OS because of early distant metastasis.

Systemic Therapy

There have been limited studies of adjuvant systemic therapy in patients with MM. A randomized phase II study in China evaluated observation versus high-dose interferon (IFN)-α-2b (HDI) versus combination chemotherapy with temozolomide and cisplatin in patients with stage I/II MM found significant survival benefits with adjuvant chemotherapy.[19] This finding was repeated in a phase III study comparing adjuvant chemotherapy with HDI.[20] Although the results of these studies are impressive, they need to be shown in a broader patient population to be considered standard of care for Western patients.

Metastatic disease has historically been treated with combinations of cytotoxic chemotherapy and immune-modulating agents extrapolated from studies of NACM. A retrospective, single-institution cohort study with advanced and unresectable MM found that cytotoxic therapy represented 82% and 51% of first-line and second-line regimens, respectively, with response rates up to 10% and median OS less than a year.[21]

Given the unique molecular features of MM, targeted therapies have been evaluated with the hope of improving patient outcomes. Although BRAF mutations are seen with far less frequency in mucosal disease compared with NACM, patients with BRAF-mutated MM treated with inhibitors have seen modest benefits. Given the high incidence of KIT mutations, treatment with imatinib mesylate, a small molecular inhibitor of KIT, was evaluated in an unselected populations but was ineffective.[22] Subsequent studies in selected patient populations found partial response rates between 23% and 54%,[23,24] although larger studies would be needed to define the true therapeutic efficacy.

Immune checkpoint blockade (ICB) emerged as an effective and well-tolerated therapeutic option for NACM. A previous multicenter study of 30 patients with advanced MM evaluated the use of ipilimumab, an inhibitor of cytotoxic T lymphocyte–associated protein 4 (CTLA-4). They found 1 patient achieving a complete response, 1 patient with a partial response, and 6 patients with stable disease. Of note, 10 patients with progression of disease did not undergo confirmatory scans per criteria, which may have confounded the results.[25] The use of ipilimumab and pembrolizumab, a PD-L1 inhibitor, in a single-institution cases series showed an objective response rate (ORR) of 11.8% with some patients experiencing durable responses.[26] A post hoc analysis of KEYNOTE-001, KEYNOTE-002, and KEYNOTE-006 evaluated pembrolizumab in patients with advanced MM and found an ORR of 19% and a median OS of 11.3 months.[27] The lagging response rates with single-agent ICB in mucosal patients prompted an investigation into the benefit of combination therapy with ipilimumab and nivolumab, a PD-L1 inhibitor. A pooled analysis of 889 patients with both MM and NACM who received either single-agent nivolumab or combination therapy showed an improved ORR (37.1% vs 23.3%) with combination treatment.[28] Although ICB has expanded the limited therapeutic options for patients with MM, further work is required to help bridge the response gaps seen in NACM.

UVEAL MELANOMA
Epidemiology and Clinical Features

Uveal melanoma (UM) is the most common primary intraocular malignancy, accounting for 85% to 95% of primary ocular malignancies and 3% to 5% of all melanoma cases.[29] These malignancies arise from melanocytes within the uveal tract, which consists of the iris, ciliary body, and choroid (**Fig. 2**).

The incidence of UM in the United States has remained stable over the last 4 decades with an age-adjusted incidence rate of 4.3 to 5.2 cases per million. Risk factors for the disease include light-colored eyes, fair skin, congenital ocular melanocytosis, dysplastic nevi, cutaneous melanoma, and BAP1 mutation.[30] Unlike NACM, it is unclear whether ultraviolet (UV) radiation exposure is a significant risk factor for UM despite many similar patient characteristics.[31]

Patients are often asymptomatic at the time of diagnosis, with lesions identified on routine eye examinations. Clinical features typically manifest as vision symptoms, including visual field loss, blurred vision, photopsia, metamorphopsia, and pain. A diagnosis can be made based on fundoscopic examination with the aid of advanced testing techniques including gonioscopy, transillumination, fluorescein angiography, ultrasonography, and optical coherence tomography.

Pathogenesis and Natural History

Mutation analysis of UM (discussed later) also diverges from that of NACM, although light-dependent mechanisms are present. An analysis of tumor initiation has also noted nonuniform distribution with predominant occurrence in the macular area consistent with dose distribution of light.[32]

Definitive treatment of the primary tumor with radiotherapy or enucleation results in low rates of local recurrence. However, despite effective local control, metastatic disease occurs in more than 50% of patients.[33] Metastatic UM involves the liver in more than 90% of cases and arises from hematologic spread. The disease's proclivity for liver metastasis has been evaluated in murine and human tumor studies, which revealed expression of cMET and CXCR4. Both receptors have been found to respond to growth factors found in the liver. Other sites of involvement for metastatic UM include the lung, bone, brain, lymph nodes, and skin.

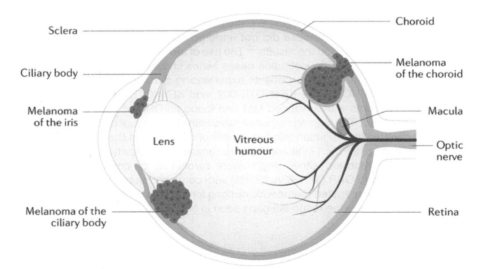

Fig. 2. Sites of uveal melanoma. (*From* Jager, M.J., Shields, C.L., Cebulla, C.M. et al. Uveal melanoma. Nat Rev Dis Primers 6, 24 (2020). https://doi.org/10.1038/s41572-020-0158-0.)

Both early and late relapses can occur, with 20% to 30% of patients dying of systemic disease within 5 years of diagnosis and 45% dying within 15 years. This pattern of recurrence has helped shape surveillance plans after local definitive treatment. In addition, prognostic markers have been identified to help determine recurrence risk and tailor surveillance regimens for individual patients. Patients harboring chromosome 3 loss and 8q rearrangements experience inferior outcomes.[34] Additional cytogenetic abnormalities, including copy number alterations in 1p, 6q, and 8p, have been shown to have higher risk for distant recurrence.[35] RNA-based gene expression assays are also commonly used to predict risk for metastatic recurrence. Patients with low metastatic risk defined as DecisionDX class 1 are maintained on active surveillance. For patients with DecisionDX class 2 disease who have an increased risk of disease recurrence, surveillance is the current standard of care; however, the evaluation of adjuvant therapies is ongoing.

Molecular Features and Immune Biology

The largest evaluation of primary UM tumors was conducted through the TCGA project, which reviewed copy number alteration, mutations, and gene and protein expression.[36] UM has molecular features that are distinct from NACM, MM, and acral lentiginous melanoma (ALM), which places the disease in a separate category. GNAQ or GNA11 mutations are found in more than 90% of cases, typically at the Q209 position.[37] For patients with wild-type GNAQ or GNA11, mutations in PLCB4 and CYSLTR2 are commonly seen and generally occur in a mutually exclusive pattern, with rare exceptions. As mentioned previously, a mutation in the BRCA1-associated protein 1 (BAP1) tumor suppressor gene found on chromosome 3 is associated with poor outcomes. BAP1 loss was found in more than 84% of metastatic tumors.[38] Somatic mutations of SF3B1 and EIF1AX occur in patients with disomy 3 and have been associated with a relatively good prognosis.[39] Categorization of UM based on distinct molecular and genetic features has led to several distinct clinical subtypes (Table 3).

A subset of high-metastasis tumors with associated angiogenesis has been shown to have TILs, predominantly composed of CD8+ T cells, macrophages, and FOXP3+ regulatory T (Treg) cells.[40] Immunosuppressive mediators have also been noted at the tumor with expression of PD-L1, transforming growth factor-β, macrophage migration inhibitor factor, and indoleamine dioxygenase-1.[41] Unlike other tumors where TIL presence indicates improved outcomes, the presence of TILs in primary UM, particularly Treg cells, has been associated with a worse prognosis.[42]

Table 3
Molecular subtypes

Metastatic Potential	mRNA GEP	Chromosome 3	Chromosome 8q	Key Mutation	Additional Mutations
Low	Class 1A	2 copies	2 copies	EIF1AX	MALAT1, LINC00645, ATM, MYC/MAX
Intermediate	Class 1B	2 copies	Partial gain	SF3B1	ZNF667-AS1, LINC00158, AKT1, p38
High	Class 2	1 copy	3 or more copies	BAP1	BANCR, LINC00152, ATM, MYC/MAX/MIZ, HIF1a, JAK/STAT, SNHG11, LINC00403, FOX1A/M1, E2F1

Abbreviations: GEP, gene expression profiling; mRNA, messenger RNA.

Therapeutic Options

Surgical management

Enucleation was the standard-of-care surgical technique for management of primary UM until the 1970s, when alternative, globe-conserving treatments started to emerge. The Collaborative Ocular Melanoma Study (COMS) was a large, prospective trial comparing enucleation with RT in patients with medium-sized choroidal melanoma.[43] The study found no difference in survival between the two groups. At present, enucleation is reserved for patients with large tumors, complete vision loss, or poor visual potential and extensive retinal detachment. Local resection with tissue conservation is technically challenging, particularly with an exoresection approach.

Radiation therapy

Multiple radiation delivery modalities are available for the treatment of primary UM. Brachytherapy is the most common RT delivery method and uses radioisotope plaques including iodine-125, cobalt-60, ruthenium-106, and palladium-103, which are sutured onto the sclera directly over the tumor to deliver focal radiation. Side effects associated with this treatment include radiation retinopathy, which is seen in approximately 50% of treated patients; optic atrophy; cataracts; vitreous hemorrhage; central retinal vein occlusion; and secondary glaucoma.[44] Charged-particle radiotherapy may also be used for medium and large tumors (>18 mm diameter or >8 mm height) or tumor locations not amenable to plaque therapy (involving the macula, optic disc, nerve, or extrascleral extension). Stereotactic photon therapy uses high doses of radiation with excellent local control rates; however, late toxicities, including chronic optic nerve atrophy, have been observed.[45] Laser photocoagulation and transpupillary thermotherapy are typically reserved for small tumors owing to higher rates of recurrence or in combination with brachytherapy, although benefits have not been consistently shown.[46] Photodynamic therapy uses a nonthermal laser that activates a photosensitive compound injected at the primary tumor, resulting in free oxygen radical generation and tissue damage.

Adjuvant therapy

Both dacarbazine, an alkylating agent, and IFN were studied in the adjuvant setting given its efficacy in NACM before the emergence of ICB; however, no survival benefit was observed.[47] Even in combination, patients with high-risk UM did not see a difference in 5-year metastasis-free survival.[48]

Additional adjuvant studies are ongoing that target the pathogenesis of metastasis using c-Met, epidermal growth factor receptor (EGFR), and insulinlike growth factor receptor 1 (IGFR1) inhibition. The use of sunitinib, a multikinase inhibitor, showed a survival benefit in the adjuvant setting compared with historical control and is currently being evaluated in a prospective, phase II study.[49] Epigenetic modifiers are also under evaluation given the role of BAP1 mutations and impaired melanocytic differentiation. Ipilimumab was evaluated recently in 84 patients for adjuvant treatment, with a median distant metastasis–free survival of 4.6 years.[50] Given the high risk for metastatic disease despite local control, meaningful adjuvant treatment remains an important area for further investigation.

For metastatic disease, treatment can be grouped into several categories, including liver-directed therapies, cytotoxic chemotherapy, immunotherapy, molecular-targeted therapies, and epigenetic modifiers. Metastatic disease has very poor outcomes, with 1-year OS of 43% from the time of the original diagnosis.[51] Liver-directed therapies include resection, radiofrequency ablation, stereotactic radiotherapy, regional chemotherapy, and embolization. The use of regional chemotherapy with fotemustine and melphalan via intrahepatic artery infusion was compared with systemic chemotherapy without improvement in OS despite differences in progression-free survival (PFS).[52]

Treatment using chemotherapy regimens adopted from NACM have shown inferior outcomes. Use of regimens containing dacarbazine, temozolomide, cisplatin, bendamustine, treosulfan, gemcitabine, and fotemustine, along with various combinations, resulted in responses ranging from 0% to 15% without significant benefits in survival.[53,54]

Checkpoint blockade has not yielded the same responses in metastatic UM as it has in advanced NACM, potentially because of the low mutational burden and immunosuppressive tumor microenvironment described previously. Single-agent ipilimumab was evaluated in large retrospective studies and several single-arm phase II studies, with ORR ranging from 0% to 8%.[55,56] Pembrolizumab was evaluated in patients who failed ipilimumab, with responses ranging from 8% to 38%, although samples sizes were very small.[57] In another study, 56 patients with metastatic UM, of whom 63% were previously treated with ipilimumab, were evaluated on programmed cell death protein 1 (PD-1) or PDL-1 antibody therapy. The study found objective tumor responses in 2 patients, with an ORR of 3.6%, median PFS of 2.6 months, and median OS of 7.6 months.[58] Studies that have evaluated the combination of ipilimumab with nivolumab are listed in **Table 4**.

Novel immune therapeutics are emerging treatments in UM. IMCgp100 is a bispecific biologic targeting the T-cell receptor and gp100, a melanocyte-associated glycoprotein present in approximately 50% of patients with UM, with clinical trials currently ongoing.

High rates of GNAQ and GNA11 mutations with downstream activation of the MAPK signaling pathway prompted studies of targeted inhibitors of this pathway. MEK inhibition, with selumetinib, was evaluated in a phase III study of patients with metastatic UM compared with cytotoxic chemotherapy (dacarbazine or temozolomide). Despite showing improved PFS with selumetinib, there was no significant difference in OS.[59] However, there was significant crossover from the chemotherapy arm to selumetinib at the time of progression, which may have confounded the results.

Although overall mutation burden is low in UM with few somatic variants, epigenetic regulation through DNA methylation or histone acetylation may be a pathway for oncogenesis. Bromodomain and extraterminal (BET) protein inhibition targets the BET family of proteins, including BRD2-4 and bromodomain testis associated (BRDT), which act as epigenetic regulators directing DNA replication and transcriptional elongation. Multiple histone deacetylase (HDAC) inhibitors have shown antitumor activity, with growth arrest and apoptosis in preclinical models.[60] Evaluation

Table 4					
Ipilimumab and nivolumab in metastatic uveal melanoma					
Study	Phase	N	RR (%)	PFS (mo)	OS (mo)
Najjar Y et al[63]	NA	66	11	2.7 (RECIST)	13.6
Heppt et al,[64] 2019	NA	64	15.6	3.0 (RECIST)	16.1
Piulats J et al[66] (GEM) [X]	II	52	12	2.8 (RECIST)	14.3
Pelster et al[65] 2019	II	35	17	6.3 (irRC)	19.2

Abbreviations: NA, not available; RR, relative risk.
Data from Refs.[63–65]

of epigenetics modifiers both as single agents and in combination with ICB is ongoing.

SUMMARY

Extracutaneous melanoma, including MM and UM, is characterized by an aggressive natural history, molecular diversity, and limited efficacy of current treatment regimens. Mucosal disease shares molecular and immunologic features similar to ALM. Despite these similarities, patients with ALM tend to have better responses to treatments such as ICB. In addition, local treatment of both mucosal and uveal disease does not seem to influence OS. Further studies of systemic therapy in the adjuvant setting need to be prioritized to help improve patient outcomes. For uveal disease, the unique molecular profile has continued to spur development of novel therapeutic agents and remains an open frontier for investigation.

CLINICS CARE POINTS

- ECM includes MM and UM, which are both characterized by aggressive natural histories and poor prognosis despite local treatment
- MM typically afflicts glabrous surfaces of the head and neck, and anorectal and vulvovaginal regions
- Given limited benefits in OS with surgical resection and/or radiation, radical surgeries are generally discouraged
- Systemic treatments with chemotherapy, ICB, and targeted therapies have seen small benefits in patients with MM
- UM risk factors are generally similar to risk factors for cutaneous melanoma, although the pathogenesis seems to be different (eg, unrelated to UV radiation–associated mutational damage)
- GNAQ or GNA11, PLCB4, and CYSLTR2 mutations are commonly seen in UM
- Risk stratification with DecisionDX based on genomic studies has helped identify high-risk patients and tailor surveillance programs
- Systemic treatments include cytotoxic chemotherapy, ICB, liver-directed therapies, targeted therapies, and epigenetic modifiers

DISCLOSURE

Authors have nothing to disclose.

REFERENCES

1. McLaughlin CC, Wu XC, Jemal A, et al. Incidence of noncutaneous melanomas in the U.S. Cancer 2005;103(5):1000–7.
2. Chang AE, Karnell LH, Menck HR. The National Cancer Data Base report on cutaneous and noncutaneous melanoma: a summary of 84,836 cases from the past decade. The American College of Surgeons Commission on Cancer and the American Cancer Society. Cancer 1998;83(8):1664–78.
3. Chan KK, Chan RC, Ho RS, et al. Clinical Patterns of Melanoma in Asians: 11-Year Experience in a Tertiary Referral Center. Ann Plast Surg 2016;77(Suppl 1):S6–11.
4. Altieri L, Wong MK, Peng DH, et al. Mucosal melanomas in the racially diverse population of California. J Am Acad Dermatol 2017;76(2):250–7.
5. Hahn HM, Lee KG, Choi W, et al. An updated review of mucosal melanoma: Survival meta-analysis. Mol Clin Oncol 2019;11(2):116–26.

6. Carvajal RD, Spencer SA, Lydiatt W. Mucosal melanoma: a clinically and biologically unique disease entity. J Natl Compr Canc Netw 2012;10(3):345–56.
7. Altieri L, Eguchi M, Peng DH, et al. Predictors of mucosal melanoma survival in a population-based setting. J Am Acad Dermatol 2019;81(1):136–42.e2.
8. Furney SJ, Turajlic S, Stamp G, et al. Genome sequencing of mucosal melanomas reveals that they are driven by distinct mechanisms from cutaneous melanoma. J Pathol 2013;230(3):261–9.
9. Hayward NK, Wilmott JS, Waddell N, et al. Whole-genome landscapes of major melanoma subtypes. Nature 2017;545(7653):175–80.
10. Newell F, Kong Y, Wilmott JS, et al. Whole-genome landscape of mucosal melanoma reveals diverse drivers and therapeutic targets. Nat Commun 2019;10(1): 3163.
11. Nassar KW, Tan AC. The mutational landscape of mucosal melanoma. Semin Cancer Biol 2020;61:139–48.
12. Carvajal RD, Antonescu CR, Wolchok JD, et al. KIT as a therapeutic target in metastatic melanoma. JAMA 2011;305(22):2327–34.
13. Kong Y, Si L, Li Y, et al. Analysis of mTOR Gene Aberrations in Melanoma Patients and Evaluation of Their Sensitivity to PI3K-AKT-mTOR Pathway Inhibitors. Clin Cancer Res 2016;22(4):1018–27.
14. Sheng X, Kong Y, Li Y, et al. GNAQ and GNA11 mutations occur in 9.5% of mucosal melanoma and are associated with poor prognosis. Eur J Cancer 2016;65:156–63.
15. Xu L, Cheng Z, Cui C, et al. Frequent genetic aberrations in the cell cycle related genes in mucosal melanoma indicate the potential for targeted therapy. J Transl Med 2019;17(1):245.
16. Kaunitz GJ, Cottrell TR, Lilo M, et al. Melanoma subtypes demonstrate distinct PD-L1 expression profiles. Lab Invest 2017;97(9):1063–71.
17. Hanna E, DeMonte F, Ibrahim S, et al. Endoscopic resection of sinonasal cancers with and without craniotomy: oncologic results. Arch Otolaryngol Head Neck Surg 2009;135(12):1219–24.
18. Matsuda A, Miyashita M, Matsumoto S, et al. Abdominoperineal resection provides better local control but equivalent overall survival to local excision of anorectal malignant melanoma: a systematic review. Ann Surg 2015;261(4):670–7.
19. Lian B, Si L, Cui C, et al. Phase II randomized trial comparing high-dose IFN-α2b with temozolomide plus cisplatin as systemic adjuvant therapy for resected mucosal melanoma. Clin Cancer Res 2013;19(16):4488–98.
20. Lian B, Cui C, Song X, et al. Phase III randomized, multicenter trial comparing high-dose IFN-a2b with temozolomide plus cisplatin as adjuvant therapy for resected mucosal melanoma. J Clin Oncol 2018;36(15_suppl):9589.
21. Shoushtari AN, Bluth MJ, Goldman DA, et al. Clinical features and response to systemic therapy in a historical cohort of advanced or unresectable mucosal melanoma. Melanoma Res 2017;27(1):57–64.
22. Kim KB, Eton O, Davis DW, et al. Phase II trial of imatinib mesylate in patients with metastatic melanoma. Br J Cancer 2008;99(5):734–40.
23. Guo J, Si L, Kong Y, et al. Phase II, open-label, single-arm trial of imatinib mesylate in patients with metastatic melanoma harboring c-Kit mutation or amplification. J Clin Oncol 2011;29(21):2904–9.
24. Hodi FS, Corless CL, Giobbie-Harder A, et al. Imatinib for melanomas harboring mutationally activated or amplified KIT arising on mucosal, acral, and chronically sun-damaged skin. J Clin Oncol 2013;31(26):3182–90.

25. Postow MA, Luke JJ, Bluth MJ, et al. Ipilimumab for patients with advanced mucosal melanoma. Oncologist 2013;18(6):726–32.

26. Kuo JC. Immune checkpoint inhibitors in the treatment of advanced mucosal melanoma. Melanoma Manag 2017;4(3):161–7.

27. Shoushtari AN, Munhoz RR, Kuk D, et al. The efficacy of anti-PD-1 agents in acral and mucosal melanoma. Cancer 2016;122(21):3354–62.

28. D'Angelo SP, Larkin J, Sosman JA, et al. Efficacy and Safety of Nivolumab Alone or in Combination With Ipilimumab in Patients With Mucosal Melanoma: A Pooled Analysis. J Clin Oncol 2017;35(2):226–35.

29. Aronow ME, Topham AK, Singh AD. Uveal Melanoma: 5-Year Update on Incidence, Treatment, and Survival (SEER 1973-2013). Ocul Oncol Pathol 2018; 4(3):145–51.

30. Walpole S, Pritchard AL, Cebulla CM, et al. Comprehensive Study of the Clinical Phenotype of Germline BAP1 Variant-Carrying Families Worldwide. J Natl Cancer Inst 2018;110(12):1328–41.

31. Shah CP, Weis E, Lajous M, et al. Intermittent and chronic ultraviolet light exposure and uveal melanoma: a meta-analysis. Ophthalmology 2005;112(9): 1599–607.

32. Singh AD, Rennie IG, Seregard S, et al. Sunlight exposure and pathogenesis of uveal melanoma. Surv Ophthalmol 2004;49(4):419–28.

33. Kujala E, Mäkitie T, Kivelä T. Very long-term prognosis of patients with malignant uveal melanoma. Invest Ophthalmol Vis Sci 2003;44(11):4651–9.

34. Versluis M, de Lange MJ, van Pelt SI, et al. Digital PCR validates 8q dosage as prognostic tool in uveal melanoma. PLoS One 2015;10(3):e0116371.

35. Shain AH, Bagger MM, Yu R, et al. The genetic evolution of metastatic uveal melanoma. Nat Genet 2019;51(7):1123–30.

36. Robertson AG, Shih J, Yau C, et al. Integrative Analysis Identifies Four Molecular and Clinical Subsets in Uveal Melanoma. Cancer Cell 2017;32(2):204–20.e15.

37. Shoushtari AN, Carvajal RD. GNAQ and GNA11 mutations in uveal melanoma. Melanoma Res 2014;24(6):525–34.

38. Harbour JW, Onken MD, Roberson ED, et al. Frequent mutation of BAP1 in metastasizing uveal melanomas. Science 2010;330(6009):1410–3.

39. Martin M, Maßhöfer L, Temming P, et al. Exome sequencing identifies recurrent somatic mutations in EIF1AX and SF3B1 in uveal melanoma with disomy 3. Nat Genet 2013;45(8):933–6.

40. Bronkhorst IH, Vu TH, Jordanova ES, et al. Different Subsets of Tumor-Infiltrating Lymphocytes Correlate with Macrophage Influx and Monosomy 3 in Uveal Melanoma. Invest Ophthalmol Vis Sci 2012;53(9):5370–8.

41. Nagarkatti-Gude N, Bronkhorst IH, van Duinen SG, et al. Cytokines and Chemokines in the Vitreous Fluid of Eyes with Uveal Melanoma. Invest Ophthalmol Vis Sci 2012;53(11):6748–55.

42. Lagouros E, Salomao D, Thorland E, et al. Infiltrative T regulatory cells in enucleated uveal melanomas. Trans Am Ophthalmol Soc 2009;107:223–8.

43. Hawkins BS. The Collaborative Ocular Melanoma Study (COMS) randomized trial of pre-enucleation radiation of large choroidal melanoma: IV. Ten-year mortality findings and prognostic factors. COMS report number 24. Am J Ophthalmol 2004;138(6):936–51.

44. Char DH, Castro JR, Quivey JM, et al. Uveal melanoma radiation. 125I brachytherapy versus helium ion irradiation. Ophthalmology 1989;96(12):1708–15.

45. Akbaba S, Foerster R, Nicolay NH, et al. Linear accelerator-based stereotactic fractionated photon radiotherapy as an eye-conserving treatment for uveal melanoma. Radiat Oncol 2018;13(1):140.
46. Marinkovic M, Horeweg N, Fiocco M, et al. Ruthenium-106 brachytherapy for choroidal melanoma without transpupillary thermotherapy: Similar efficacy with improved visual outcome. Eur J Cancer 2016;68:106–13.
47. Lane AM, Egan KM, Harmon D, et al. Adjuvant interferon therapy for patients with uveal melanoma at high risk of metastasis. Ophthalmology 2009;116(11): 2206–12.
48. Binkley E, Triozzi PL, Rybicki L, et al. A prospective trial of adjuvant therapy for high-risk uveal melanoma: assessing 5-year survival outcomes. Br J Ophthalmol 2020;104(4):524–8.
49. Valsecchi ME, Orloff M, Sato R, et al. Adjuvant Sunitinib in High-Risk Patients with Uveal Melanoma: Comparison with Institutional Controls. Ophthalmology 2018; 125(2):210–7.
50. Fountain E, Bassett R, Cain S, et al. Adjuvant Ipilimumab in High-Risk Uveal Melanoma. Cancers (Basel) 2019;11(2):152.
51. Khoja L, Atenafu EG, Suciu S, et al. Meta-analysis in metastatic uveal melanoma to determine progression free and overall survival benchmarks: an international rare cancers initiative (IRCI) ocular melanoma study. Ann Oncol 2019;30(8): 1370–80.
52. Hughes MS, Zager J, Faries M, et al. Results of a Randomized Controlled Multicenter Phase III Trial of Percutaneous Hepatic Perfusion Compared with Best Available Care for Patients with Melanoma Liver Metastases. Ann Surg Oncol 2016;23(4):1309–19.
53. Spagnolo F, Grosso M, Picasso V, et al. Treatment of metastatic uveal melanoma with intravenous fotemustine. Melanoma Res 2013;23(3):196–8.
54. Schmittel A, Schmidt-Hieber M, Martus P, et al. A randomized phase II trial of gemcitabine plus treosulfan versus treosulfan alone in patients with metastatic uveal melanoma. Ann Oncol 2006;17(12):1826–9.
55. Piulats Rodriguez JM, Ochoa de Olza M, Codes M, et al. Phase II study evaluating ipilimumab as a single agent in the first-line treatment of adult patients (Pts) with metastatic uveal melanoma (MUM): The GEM-1 trial. J Clin Oncol 2014;32(15_suppl):9033.
56. Zimmer L, Vaubel J, Mohr P, et al. Phase II DeCOG-study of ipilimumab in pretreated and treatment-naïve patients with metastatic uveal melanoma. PLoS One 2015;10(3):e0118564.
57. Karydis I, Chan PY, Wheater M, et al. Clinical activity and safety of Pembrolizumab in Ipilimumab pre-treated patients with uveal melanoma. Oncoimmunology 2016;5(5):e1143997.
58. Algazi AP, Tsai KK, Shoushtari AN, et al. Clinical outcomes in metastatic uveal melanoma treated with PD-1 and PD-L1 antibodies. Cancer 2016;122(21): 3344–53.
59. Carvajal RD, Sosman JA, Quevedo JF, et al. Effect of selumetinib vs chemotherapy on progression-free survival in uveal melanoma: a randomized clinical trial. JAMA 2014;311(23):2397–405.
60. Moschos MM, Dettoraki M, Androudi S, et al. The Role of Histone Deacetylase Inhibitors in Uveal Melanoma: Current Evidence. Anticancer Res 2018;38(7): 3817–24.

61. Lian B, Cui CL, Zhou L, et al. The natural history and patterns of metastases from mucosal melanoma: an analysis of 706 prospectively-followed patients. Ann Oncol 2017;28(4):868–73.
62. Patrick RJ, Fenske NA, Messina JL. Primary mucosal melanoma. J Am Acad Dermatol 2007;56(5):828–34.
63. Najjar Y, Navrazhina K, Bhatia R, et al. Outcomes for patients with metastatic uveal melanoma (MUM) treated with ipilimumab and nivolumab (cIN): a multicenter, retrospective study. SMR Congress 2018 Abstracts. Pigment Cell Melanoma Res 2019;32(1):92–172.
64. Heppt MV, Amaral T, Kähler KC, et al. Combined immune checkpoint blockade for metastatic uveal melanoma: a retrospective, multi-center study. J Immunother Cancer 2019;7(1):299.
65. Pelster M, Gruschkus SK, Bassett R, et al. Phase II study of ipilimumab and nivolumab (ipi/nivo) in metastatic uveal melanoma (UM). J Clin Oncol 2019; 37(15_suppl):9522.
66. Piulats Rodriguez JM, De La Cruz Merino L, Espinosa E, et al. Phase II multicenter, single arm, open label study of Nivolumab in combination with Ipilimumab in untreated patients with metastatic uveal melanoma (GEM1402). Annals of Oncology 2018;29(suppl_8):viii4442–66.

Immune Checkpoint Therapies for Melanoma

Elizabeth I. Buchbinder, MD

KEYWORDS

- Immune checkpoint inhibition • Melanoma • Immunotherapy

KEY POINTS

- Immune checkpoint inhibitors targeting cytotoxic T-lymphocyte–associated protein 4 and programmed cell death protein 1 are approved for the treatment of advanced melanoma alone and in combination.
- These agents are approved for use in high-risk resected stage III melanoma in the adjuvant setting.
- Clinical trials testing the combination of immune checkpoint inhibition with other therapies and novel immunotherapies continue.

INTRODUCTION

Before 2011 the world of melanoma treatment was a relatively bleak place. Treatment options for metastatic melanoma consisted of high-dose interleukin-2 or chemotherapy such as dacarbazine. High-dose interleukin-2 can lead to durable responses for a small number of patients.[1] However, high-dose interleukin-2 is extremely toxic and requires inpatient administration with close monitoring. Dacarbazine and other chemotherapy regimens have limited activity in melanoma treatment with roughly 20% response rates. In addition, for those patients who do respond to chemotherapy the responses are generally of limited duration.[2,3]

The adjuvant therapy space for high-risk melanoma was not much more promising at that time. Adjuvant therapy consisted of high-dose interferon alfa-2b or pegylated interferon.[4–6] These therapies are limited by their high rate of toxicity and low benefit. Almost all patients treated with the different forms of interferon experience flulike syndrome, depression, and severe fatigue. Efforts to better uncover the optimal way to give adjuvant therapies in melanoma were limited by the small benefits observed.[7]

Although therapies for melanoma were limited, it was known that the immune system played an important role in the detection and control of melanoma. Scientific advances have led to a better understanding of immune system function and the

Dana-Farber Cancer Institute, 450 Brookline Avenue, Boston, MA 02481, USA
E-mail address: Elizabeth_buchbinder@dfci.harvard.edu

Hematol Oncol Clin N Am 35 (2021) 99–109
https://doi.org/10.1016/j.hoc.2020.08.013
0889-8588/21/© 2020 Elsevier Inc. All rights reserved.

hemonc.theclinics.com

complex signaling between the cells involved in mounting an anticancer immune response. From this knowledge the world of immune checkpoint therapy grew and began a new and more hopeful era in the world of melanoma therapy.

IMMUNE CHECKPOINT INHIBITION

To function properly the immune system must be able to identify foreign substances while still recognizing what is self. Part of this process is recognition and binding of the T-cell receptor (TCR) with an antigen displayed in the major histocompatibility complex (MHC) on the surface of an antigen-presenting cell (APC). Circulating T cells are exposed to professional APCs displaying foreign antigens (infection) or mutated self-proteins (malignancy).

To prevent autoimmunity, numerous immune checkpoint pathways regulate activation of T cells at multiple steps during an immune response.[8,9] Some of these checkpoints are involved in activation of T cells. One such protein, B7, is expressed on the surface of APCs, and its interaction with CD28 expressed on T cells leads to T-cell activation.

Other proteins are involved in downregulation of the immune response. Cytotoxic T-lymphocyte–associated protein 4 (CTLA-4) is expressed on activated T cells and interacts with B7 on APCs leading to T-cell inhibition.[10,11] There is evidence that CTLA-4 signaling is also involved early in the course of T-cell development.[12] In vivo studies demonstrated that antibodies that block CTLA-4 led to increased T-cell activation and increased immune response against tumors, which was confirmed in vitro.[13,14]

Another inhibitory checkpoint involves the interaction of programmed death protein 1 (PD-1) and its ligands PD-L1 and PD-L2. PD-1 is a member of the CD28 family and involved in immune inhibition and associated with T-cell exhaustion.[15–17] PD-1 binds to PD-L1 and PD-L2, leading to limitation of effector T-cell responses.[18]

Although CTLA-4 and PD-1 are currently the most targeted of the immune checkpoint interactions, there are numerous stimulatory and inhibitory interactions that occur within the immune system. There are continued efforts to target these novel checkpoints and continue to better understand the signaling that occurs within the immune system. Studies have demonstrated differences in the mechanism by which CTLA-4 and PD-1 bring about changes in T-cell activation.[19] Differences in these checkpoint pathways provide opportunities for combination therapies.

Tumors, which would normally be recognized by T cells, have developed ways to evade the host immune system by taking advantage of these immune checkpoint pathways. Tumors express PD-L1 leading to T-cell inhibition. In addition, they have been shown to downregulate MHC class I on tumor cells and recruit myeloid-derived suppressor cells and regulatory T cells that inhibit immune activity.[20] Overcoming this immune inhibition has huge potential in oncology.

CYTOTOXIC T-LYMPHOCYTE–ASSOCIATED PROTEIN 4 INHIBITION (IPILIMUMAB)

In vivo and in vitro evidence of antitumor effect from CTLA-4 blockade led to clinical trials of anti-CTLA-4 antibodies in patients with advanced melanoma.[21,22] It was observed that a selection of patients responded to treatment with CTLA-4 blockade and that responses were durable, continuing even after therapy was stopped. These early signs of activity in melanoma led to the development of ipilimumab, an anti-CTLA-4 Ab.

The first randomized phase 3 study of ipilimumab enrolled 676 patients who were HLA-A*0201 positive and had unresectable stage III or IV melanoma. Patients were randomized in a 3:1:1 ratio to receive ipilimumab plus gp100 (a peptide vaccine), ipilimumab alone, or gp100 alone. This study completely revolutionized the treatment of melanoma when it demonstrated an overall survival benefit in those patients treated with ipilimumab over those treated with gp100 alone with median overall survival of 10.0, 10.1, and 6.4 months in each of the respective groups.[23]

The benefit of ipilimumab was confirmed in a phase 3 study comparing ipilimumab combined with dacarbazine versus dacarbazine alone. This study enrolled 502 patients and again demonstrated an improved overall survival in those patients who received ipilimumab at 11.2 months in the combination group versus 9.1 months in the dacarbazine alone group.[24]

In addition to dramatically changing the treatment landscape for advanced melanoma, these studies also revealed new patterns of response to immunotherapy and novel toxicity patterns. Atypical response patterns included pseudoprogression with patients having initial disease growth on imaging followed by regression. This observation of pseudoprogression led to the development of immune-related response criteria or iRECIST for clinical trials to avoid stopping a promising drug too early in immunotherapy clinical trials.[25]

The toxicities associated with ipilimumab are also very different and follow a very different pattern from traditional chemotherapy. Autoimmune toxicities including colitis, hypophysitis, hepatitis, pancreatitis, and many others were documented. Treatment of these toxicities involves immunosuppression with steroids or other immune suppression. The pattern of these toxicities is also novel, with severe side effects arising weeks to months after patients start on therapy.[26]

Ipilimumab was the first therapy to demonstrate a survival benefit in the treatment of advanced melanoma and became the standard therapy from which subsequent therapies were developed.

PROGRAMMED CELL DEATH PROTEIN 1 INHIBITION (NIVOLUMAB AND PEMBROLIZUMAB)

Blockade of PD-1 to overcome immune resistance became an active field of study in melanoma with 2 antibodies developed almost simultaneously. Nivolumab and pembrolizumab are antibodies with direct activity on PD-1.

Nivolumab was initially tested in a phase I study that enrolled patients with melanoma as well as non–small cell lung cancer, castrate-resistant prostate cancer, renal cell carcinoma, or colorectal cancer. A total of 296 patients were enrolled, and a 28% response rate was observed in the 94 patients with advanced melanoma. In addition, the rates of toxicity were low with only 14% grade 3 or 4 drug-related adverse events.[27]

Pembrolizumab was initially tested in 135 patients with advanced melanoma with a response rate of 38%. In addition, the responses were observed to be durable in most of the patients. The adverse events were overall predominantly grade 1 or 2.[28]

Phase III trials of both drugs moved forward in advanced melanoma. Nivolumab was compared with chemotherapy in a study of 405 patients with melanoma with advanced disease that was refractory to ipilimumab. Patients on this study were randomized 2:1 in favor of nivolumab and the response rate observed was 31.7% in the nivolumab group as compared with 10.6% in the chemotherapy group.[29] Another study looked at patients with advanced melanoma without BRAF mutation who were untreated. This study randomized 418 patients to nivolumab or dacarbazine. The response rate was 40% in the nivolumab group versus 13.9% in the dacarbazine group. In addition, this trial demonstrated an overall survival benefit with a 1-year overall survival rate of 72.9% in the nivolumab group versus 42.1% in the dacarbazine group.[30] Toxicity rates on these studies were similarly favorable to earlier trials.

Pembrolizumab was evaluated in a phase 3 study that compared 2 dosing regimens of pembrolizumab against ipilimumab. A total of 834 patients with advanced melanoma were enrolled and randomized in a 1:1:1 ratio. The overall response rates were 33.7% and 32.9% on the 2 pembrolizumab dosing groups as compared with 11.9% on the ipilimumab groups. The 12-month survival rates were 74.1% and 68.4% in the pembrolizumab groups as compared with 58.2% in the ipilimumab group. Toxicity was low with 13.3% and 10.1% of patients in the pembrolizumab groups experiencing grade 3 to 5 toxicity.[31]

These studies established nivolumab and pembrolizumab as standard treatment options for metastatic melanoma in the front line or after other cancer-directed therapies. In addition, they demonstrated a favorable toxicity profile with rare but significant autoimmune side effects.

COMBINATION IMMUNE CHECKPOINT INHIBITION (IPILIMUMAB/NIVOLUMAB)

Early observations demonstrated differences between CTLA-4 inhibition and PD-1 inhibition. The mechanism by which both receptors regulated T-cell activation were noted to be different.[19] In addition, the location of activity for these different receptors suggested different roles they play with more CTLA-4 signaling in the lymph node and more PD-1 signaling in tissue or tumor.[32] Findings such as these supported possible synergy of these treatments and the concept of combining or sequencing ipilimumab and nivolumab in the treatment of advanced melanoma.

To evaluate for possible synergy 945 patients with previously untreated unresectable stage III or IV melanoma were enrolled and randomized in a 1:1:1 fashion to nivolumab alone, nivolumab-plus-ipilimumab, or ipilimumab alone. This study demonstrated improved progression-free survival and response rates in the combination ipilimumab and nivolumab group. The median progression-free survival was 6.9 months in the nivolumab group, 11.5 months in the nivolumab-plus-ipilimumab group, and 2.9 months in the ipilimumab group. The response rates were noted to be 43.7% in the nivolumab group, 57.6% in the nivolumab-plus-ipilimumab group, and 19% in the ipilimumab group. However, there was note of much higher toxicity in the nivolumab-plus-ipilimumab group with a 55% incidence of grade 3 or 4 adverse events.[33]

Five-year survival numbers were published for the combination, which demonstrated that the PFS and response rate benefit observed with ipilimumab-plus-nivolumab translated into a survival benefit. The 5-year overall survival with ipilimumab-plus-nivolumab group was found to be 52%, in the nivolumab-alone group it was 44%, and in the ipilimumab alone group it was 26%. This study also evaluated subgroups including PD-L1 status with no evidence that this was a predictive marker of response in this population.[34]

Another approach explored was the sequential administration of nivolumab and ipilimumab with a planned switch after 12 weeks of therapy. This study demonstrated improved progression-free survival and overall survival in patients treated with nivolumab before ipilimumab. The 12-month overall survival was 76% in the nivolumab followed by ipilimumab group as compared with 54% in the ipilimumab followed by nivolumab group. Toxicity was noted to be similar with 50% grade 3 to 5 adverse events in the nivolumab followed by ipilimumab group and 43% in the ipilimumab followed by nivolumab group.[35]

These trials demonstrate an increased response rate and survival with combination ipilimumab and nivolumab at the cost of high autoimmune toxicity. Selecting patients most appropriate for combination therapy is important, given this high rate of side effects. A comparison of the approved immune checkpoint inhibitors is presented in **Table 1**. ·

One group for which combination ipilimumab and nivolumab has a clear benefit is patients with advanced melanoma with brain metastasis. A study enrolled 94 patients with asymptomatic brain metastasis that did not require steroids and treated them with combination ipilimumab and nivolumab. The intracranial clinical benefit rate was found to be 57% with a 56% extracranial clinical benefit rate. Adverse events were similar to that previously reported with the combination, with 55% of patients experiencing grade 3 or 4 adverse events.[36]

ADJUVANT MELANOMA IMMUNOTHERAPY

The development of immune checkpoint inhibition in the advanced melanoma setting quickly led to testing in the adjuvant setting for patients at high risk of melanoma recurrence. Patients with resected metastatic nodal disease, stage III, have frequent recurrences despite successful surgery, which renders them without evidence of disease. This population was the target for initial adjuvant therapy testing.

Ipilimumab at a dose of 10 mg/kg was evaluated in stage III melanoma after complete resection with 951 patients randomized to treatment or placebo. This trial demonstrated an improved recurrence-free survival of 40.8% for the ipilimumab group versus 30.3% for the placebo group at 5 years. In addition, there was an improvement in overall survival with a rate of 65.4% in the ipilimumab group at 5 years versus 54.4% in the placebo at 5 years. Unfortunately, the adverse event rate in patients treated with ipilimumab on this trial was 54.1% grade 3 or 4 adverse events with 41.6% severe immune-related adverse events.[37] Of note the dose used in this trial was 10 mg/kg of ipilimumab, which is more than 3 times the standard dosing of ipilimumab 3 mg/kg used in the metastatic setting.

Nivolumab was evaluated in patients with stage IIIB, IIIC, or IV melanoma following complete resection in a phase 3 randomized trial. In this trial patients were randomized to nivolumab at standard dosing or ipilimumab at the 10 mg/kg adjuvant dosing. A total of 906 patients were enrolled and treated. The 1-year recurrence-free survival was 70.5% in the nivolumab group and 60.8% in the ipilimumab group. In addition, toxicity was far lower in the nivolumab group with only 14.4% grade 3 or 4 treatment-related adverse events as compared with 45.9% in the ipilimumab group,[38] and this led to nivolumab replacing ipilimumab for the treatment of high-risk stage III melanoma patients in the adjuvant setting.

Table 1
Comparison of approved immune checkpoint inhibition in advanced melanoma

Immunotherapy	Response Rate (%)	Median PFS (mo)	Median OS (mo)	Grade 3–4 Toxicity (%)
Ipilimumab[23]	11	2–3	10–11	10–15
Nivolumab[29,30,33]	32–40	7	37	14
Pembrolizumab[31]	32	8.4	33	13
Ipilimumab and nivolumab[33]	58	11.5	>60	55

Pembrolizumab was evaluated in completely resected stage III patients in a randomized trial versus placebo. A total of 1019 patients were enrolled and treated on this trial. The 1-year recurrence-free survival rate was 75.4% for the pembrolizumab group versus 61.0% for the placebo group. The rate of grade 3 to 5 treatment-related adverse events was only 14.7% in the pembrolizumab group.[39] With this study pembrolizumab became another option for the adjuvant treatment of patients with high-risk, resected stage III melanoma.

These studies have established PD-1 inhibition with nivolumab or pembrolizumab as the immunotherapy of choice for patients with resected melanoma with evidence of disease in the lymph node, stage III melanoma. There are studies underway to determine if there is similar benefit for those patients with resected stage II melanoma and patients with a thick primary melanoma but no evidence of lymph node involvement. Patients with resected stage III melanoma that harbors a BRAF V600E or V600K mutations can also be treated with adjuvant targeted therapy with combination BRAF and MEK inhibition (dabrafenib and trametinib).

NEOADJUVANT MELANOMA IMMUNOTHERAPY

As immunotherapy established itself as an effective therapy for the prevention of recurrence of high-risk melanoma, the question of best timing emerged. One hypothesis was that a more effective immune response might be generated against a nodal metastasis before resection. In addition, starting effective therapy earlier in the course of treatment, as opposed to waiting until after surgical resection, might lead to increased long-term benefit. Based on this neoadjuvant immunotherapy has been explored in some small studies and is being explored further in larger phase 3 studies.

One trial of neoadjuvant PD-1 inhibition with a single dose of pembrolizumab before surgery demonstrated a 30% complete or near-complete pathologic response rate as well as 2-year PFS of 63% suggesting benefit.[40] Other trials of PD-1 inhibition with nivolumab or pembrolizumab also demonstrated response and pathologic complete response rates in the 25% range.[41] The OpACIN-neo trial looked at different dose schedules for combining ipilimumab and nivolumab in the neoadjuvant setting and observed rates of radiologic response ranging from 35% to 63% among the different groups and pathologic responses ranging 65% to 80% with the ipilimumab, 1 mg/kg, and nivolumab, 3 mg/kg, being determined to be the most tolerable with only 20% grade 3 to 4 immune-related adverse events.[42]

Further study of immune checkpoint therapy in the neoadjuvant setting for melanoma is ongoing and has the potential to define another area of benefit for these therapies.

OTHER IMMUNE CHECKPOINT INHIBITOR COMBINATIONS AND FUTURE DIRECTIONS

Given the success of immune checkpoint inhibition in melanoma, there have been numerous studies of immune checkpoint inhibition in combination with chemotherapy, targeted therapy, other immunotherapies, or novel drugs. There have also been trials combining immunotherapy with nonpharmacologic treatments such as radiation or cryoablation. The goal of these studies has been to improve responses and survival in melanoma while also lowering the rates of severe autoimmune toxicities.

BRAF- and MEK-targeted therapy in patients whose melanoma harbors a BRAF V600E or K mutation has high efficacy in advanced melanoma; however relapses are common. BRAF therapy has been associated with increased PD-L1 expression and CD8+ T-cell infiltrate, suggesting possible synergy between targeted therapy and immunotherapy.[43] Based on these data there have been trials examining the combination of targeted therapy with BRAF/MEK inhibition and PD-1 inhibition,[44,45] and larger trials are ongoing. These trials will help to determine if these therapies synergize or if they are just as effective when given sequentially. In addition, toxicity of combination regimens will need to be evaluated.

GM-CSF was combined with ipilimumab with an interesting result. Overall survival was improved with the combination of GM-CSF and ipilimumab but progression-free survival was not. It was found that the grade 3 to 5 treatment-related adverse event rate was much lower in the combination group at 44.9% as compared with the ipilimumab-alone group at 58.3%.[46] Based on this a trial combining granulocyte-macrophage colony-stimulating factor (GM-CSF) with ipilimumab and nivolumab has been enrolling through Eastern Cooperative Oncology Group and Southwest Oncology Group.

Talimogene laherparepvec (T-VEC) is a modified herpes simplex type 1–derived oncolytic immunotherapy, which selectively replicates within tumors and produces GM-CSF. Trials of T-VEC alone demonstrated a 16.3% durable response rate greater than 6 months.[47] A trial combining T-VEC with ipilimumab demonstrated a 39% response rate for the combination with responses observed beyond injected lesions.[48] Trials with T-VEC and immune checkpoint inhibition are ongoing. In addition, numerous other intratumoral injections including other viruses, plasmids, TLR agonists, and others are in development in combination with immune checkpoint inhibition.

Vaccines have been a very active area of research in melanoma given the immunogenicity of the tumors. Recent efforts have focused on neoantigen vaccines to improve immunogenicity and tumor specificity. Early trials have demonstrated development of neoantigen-specific T cells in response to vaccines.[49] Trials looking at clinical activity of numerous different vaccine approaches in combination with immune checkpoint inhibition in the metastatic and adjuvant setting are ongoing.

The trafficking and infiltration of immune cells into tumors are important steps in the development of an immune response. A study combining ipilimumab and bevacizumab, vascular endothelial growth factor (VEGF) inhibition, demonstrated increased immune infiltrate in patients treated with the combination over those treated with ipilimumab alone. Increased CD3+, CD8+, and CD163+ T cells infiltrating into tumors were observed. In addition, an impressive disease control rate of 67.4% was observed in 46 patients with metastatic melanoma treated with the combination.[50] Studies of different combinations of immune checkpoint blockade with VEGF inhibition or other antiangiogenic drugs are ongoing.

There is a huge range of activating and inhibiting immune modulatory receptors that have been uncovered. Activating receptors are being targeted in trials with agonistic antibodies that include such targets as CD28, OX40, GITR, and CD137. On the other end there continue to be efforts targeting inhibitory receptors with blocking antibodies. Targets under exploration include TIM-3, VISTA, and LAG-3.[51]

SUMMARY

Immune checkpoint inhibitors have revolutionized the treatment of melanoma. Ipilimumab, which targets CTLA-4, is approved for the use in advanced melanoma and in combination with PD-1 inhibition. PD-1 inhibition with nivolumab or pembrolizumab is approved for the use in advanced melanoma alone and in combination with CTLA-4 inhibition. In addition, PD-1 and CTLA-4 inhibition are approved for the adjuvant treatment of patients with high-risk stage III melanoma with PD-1 inhibition being preferred due to better tolerability and efficacy. These treatments are being tested in the adjuvant setting for stage II patients, in the neoadjuvant setting, and in combination with many novel agents in the advanced metastatic setting. The use of immune checkpoint inhibition is firmly established in the treatment of melanoma with the potential to continue expanding.

CLINICS CARE POINTS

- PD-1 inhibitors are approved for use in the adjuvant setting for the treatment of melanoma.
- Immune checkpoint inhibitors can be given alone or in combination for patients with advanced melanoma.
- Patients must be monitored closely for immune related side effects when treated with immune checkpoint inhibition.

DISCLOSURE

Dr E.I. Buchbinder received compensation for consulting from BMS, Trieza, Novartis, and Partner Therapeutics. She receives clinical trial support form Eli Lilly, Novartis, BMS, Genentech, and BVD.

REFERENCES

1. Atkins MB, Lotze MT, Dutcher JP, et al. High-dose recombinant interleukin 2 therapy for patients with metastatic melanoma: analysis of 270 patients treated between 1985 and 1993. J Clin Oncol 1999;17(7):2105–16.
2. Burke PJ, McCarthy WH, Milton GW. Imidazole carboxamide therapy in advanced malignant melanoma. Cancer 1971;27(3):744–50.
3. Hodi FS, Soiffer RJ, Clark J, et al. Phase II study of paclitaxel and carboplatin for malignant melanoma. Am J Clin Oncol 2002;25(3):283–6.
4. Kirkwood JM, Strawderman MH, Ernstoff MS, et al. Interferon alfa-2b adjuvant therapy of high-risk resected cutaneous melanoma: the Eastern Cooperative Oncology Group Trial EST 1684. J Clin Oncol 1996;14(1):7–17.
5. Jonasch E, Kumar UN, Linette GP, et al. Adjuvant high-dose interferon alfa-2b in patients with high-risk melanoma. Cancer J 2000;6(3):139–45.
6. Bottomley A, Coens C, Suciu S, et al. Adjuvant therapy with pegylated interferon alfa-2b versus observation in resected stage III melanoma: a phase III randomized controlled trial of health-related quality of life and symptoms by the European Organisation for Research and Treatment of Cancer Melanoma Group. J Clin Oncol 2009;27(18):2916–23.
7. Pectasides D, Dafni U, Bafaloukos D, et al. Randomized phase III study of 1 month versus 1 year of adjuvant high-dose interferon alfa-2b in patients with resected high-risk melanoma. J Clin Oncol 2009;27(6):939–44.
8. Goldrath AW, Bevan MJ. Selecting and maintaining a diverse T-cell repertoire. Nature 1999;402(6759):255–62.
9. Fife BT, Bluestone JA. Control of peripheral T-cell tolerance and autoimmunity via the CTLA-4 and PD-1 pathways. Immunol Rev 2008;224:166–82.
10. Walunas TL, Lenschow DJ, Bakker CY, et al. CTLA-4 can function as a negative regulator of T cell activation. Immunity 1994;1(5):405–13.
11. Krummel MF, Allison JP. CD28 and CTLA-4 have opposing effects on the response of T cells to stimulation. J Exp Med 1995;182(2):459–65.

12. Brunner MC, Chambers CA, Chan FK, et al. CTLA-4-Mediated inhibition of early events of T cell proliferation. J Immunol 1999;162(10):5813–20.

13. Leach DR, Krummel MF, Allison JP. Enhancement of antitumor immunity by CTLA-4 blockade. Science 1996;271(5256):1734–6.

14. van Elsas A, Hurwitz AA, Allison JP. Combination immunotherapy of B16 melanoma using anti-cytotoxic T lymphocyte-associated antigen 4 (CTLA-4) and granulocyte/macrophage colony-stimulating factor (GM-CSF)-producing vaccines induces rejection of subcutaneous and metastatic tumors accompanied by autoimmune depigmentation. J Exp Med 1999;190(3):355–66.

15. Koga N, Suzuki J, Kosuge H, et al. Blockade of the interaction between PD-1 and PD-L1 accelerates graft arterial disease in cardiac allografts. Arterioscler Thromb Vasc Biol 2004;24(11):2057–62.

16. Hirano F, Kaneko K, Tamura H, et al. Blockade of B7-H1 and PD-1 by monoclonal antibodies potentiates cancer therapeutic immunity. Cancer Res 2005;65(3):1089–96.

17. Day CL, Kaufmann DE, Kiepiela P, et al. PD-1 expression on HIV-specific T cells is associated with T-cell exhaustion and disease progression. Nature 2006;443(7109):350–4.

18. Keir ME, Butte MJ, Freeman GJ, et al. PD-1 and its ligands in tolerance and immunity. Annu Rev Immunol 2008;26:677–704.

19. Parry RV, Chemnitz JM, Frauwirth KA, et al. CTLA-4 and PD-1 receptors inhibit T-cell activation by distinct mechanisms. Mol Cell Biol 2005;25(21):9543–53.

20. Poschke I, Mougiakakos D, Kiessling R. Camouflage and sabotage: tumor escape from the immune system. Cancer Immunol Immunother 2011;60(8):1161–71.

21. Tchekmedyian S, Glaspy J, Korman A, et al. MDX-010(human anti CTLA-4): A phase I trial in malignant melanoma. Proc Am Soc Clin Oncol 2002;21 (abstr 56).

22. Maker AV, Yang JC, Sherry RM, et al. Intrapatient dose escalation of anti-CTLA-4 antibody in patients with metastatic melanoma. J Immunother 2006;29(4):455–63.

23. Hodi FS, O'Day SJ, McDermott DF, et al. Improved survival with ipilimumab in patients with metastatic melanoma. N Engl J Med 2010;363(8):711–23.

24. Robert C, Thomas L, Bondarenko I, et al. Ipilimumab plus dacarbazine for previously untreated metastatic melanoma. N Engl J Med 2011;364(26):2517–26.

25. O'Regan KN, Jagannathan JP, Ramaiya N, et al. Radiologic aspects of immune-related tumor response criteria and patterns of immune-related adverse events in patients undergoing ipilimumab therapy. AJR Am J Roentgenol 2011;197(2):W241–6.

26. Weber JS, Kahler KC, Hauschild A. Management of immune-related adverse events and kinetics of response with ipilimumab. J Clin Oncol 2012;30(21):2691–7.

27. Topalian SL, Hodi FS, Brahmer JR, et al. Safety, activity, and immune correlates of anti-PD-1 antibody in cancer. N Engl J Med 2012;366(26):2443–54.

28. Hamid O, Robert C, Daud A, et al. Safety and tumor responses with lambrolizumab (anti-PD-1) in melanoma. N Engl J Med 2013;369(2):134–44.

29. Weber JS, D'Angelo SP, Minor D, et al. Nivolumab versus chemotherapy in patients with advanced melanoma who progressed after anti-CTLA-4 treatment (CheckMate 037): a randomised, controlled, open-label, phase 3 trial. Lancet Oncol 2015;16(4):375–84.

30. Robert C, Long GV, Brady B, et al. Nivolumab in previously untreated melanoma without BRAF mutation. N Engl J Med 2015;372(4):320–30.

31. Robert C, Schachter J, Long GV, et al. Pembrolizumab versus Ipilimumab in Advanced Melanoma. N Engl J Med 2015;372(26):2521–32.

32. Ott PA, Hodi FS, Robert C. CTLA-4 and PD-1/PD-L1 blockade: new immunotherapeutic modalities with durable clinical benefit in melanoma patients. Clin Cancer Res 2013;19(19):5300–9.

33. Larkin J, Chiarion-Sileni V, Gonzalez R, et al. Combined Nivolumab and Ipilimumab or Monotherapy in Untreated Melanoma. N Engl J Med 2015;373(1):23–34.

34. Larkin J, Chiarion-Sileni V, Gonzalez R, et al. Five-Year Survival with Combined Nivolumab and Ipilimumab in Advanced Melanoma. N Engl J Med 2019; 381(16):1535–46.

35. Weber JS, Gibney G, Sullivan RJ, et al. Sequential administration of nivolumab and ipilimumab with a planned switch in patients with advanced melanoma (CheckMate 064): an open-label, randomised, phase 2 trial. Lancet Oncol 2016;17(7):943–55.

36. Tawbi HA, Forsyth PA, Algazi A, et al. Combined Nivolumab and Ipilimumab in Melanoma Metastatic to the Brain. N Engl J Med 2018;379(8):722–30.

37. Eggermont AM, Chiarion-Sileni V, Grob JJ, et al. Prolonged Survival in Stage III Melanoma with Ipilimumab Adjuvant Therapy. N Engl J Med 2016;375(19): 1845–55.

38. Weber J, Mandala M, Del Vecchio M, et al. Adjuvant Nivolumab versus Ipilimumab in Resected Stage III or IV Melanoma. N Engl J Med 2017;377(19): 1824–35.

39. Eggermont AMM, Blank CU, Mandala M, et al. Adjuvant Pembrolizumab versus Placebo in Resected Stage III Melanoma. N Engl J Med 2018;378(19):1789–801.

40. Huang AC, Orlowski RJ, Xu X, et al. A single dose of neoadjuvant PD-1 blockade predicts clinical outcomes in resectable melanoma. Nat Med 2019;25(3):454–61.

41. Amaria RN, Reddy SM, Tawbi HA, et al. Neoadjuvant immune checkpoint blockade in high-risk resectable melanoma. Nat Med 2018;24(11):1649–54.

42. Rozeman EA, Menzies AM, van Akkooi ACJ, et al. Identification of the optimal combination dosing schedule of neoadjuvant ipilimumab plus nivolumab in macroscopic stage III melanoma (OpACIN-neo): a multicentre, phase 2, randomised, controlled trial. Lancet Oncol 2019;20(7):948–60.

43. Frederick DT, Piris A, Cogdill AP, et al. BRAF inhibition is associated with enhanced melanoma antigen expression and a more favorable tumor microenvironment in patients with metastatic melanoma. Clin Cancer Res 2013;19(5): 1225–31.

44. Ascierto PA, Ferrucci PF, Fisher R, et al. Dabrafenib, trametinib and pembrolizumab or placebo in BRAF-mutant melanoma. Nat Med 2019;25(6):941–6.

45. Sullivan RJ, Hamid O, Gonzalez R, et al. Atezolizumab plus cobimetinib and vemurafenib in BRAF-mutated melanoma patients. Nat Med 2019;25(6):929–35.

46. Hodi FS, Lee S, McDermott DF, et al. Ipilimumab plus sargramostim vs ipilimumab alone for treatment of metastatic melanoma: a randomized clinical trial. JAMA 2014;312(17):1744–53.

47. Andtbacka RH, Kaufman HL, Collichio F, et al. Talimogene Laherparepvec Improves Durable Response Rate in Patients With Advanced Melanoma. J Clin Oncol 2015;33(25):2780–8.

48. Chesney J, Puzanov I, Collichio F, et al. Randomized, Open-Label Phase II Study Evaluating the Efficacy and Safety of Talimogene Laherparepvec in Combination With Ipilimumab Versus Ipilimumab Alone in Patients With Advanced, Unresectable Melanoma. J Clin Oncol 2018;36(17):1658–67.

49. Ott PA, Hu Z, Keskin DB, et al. An immunogenic personal neoantigen vaccine for patients with melanoma. Nature 2017;547(7662):217–21.
50. Hodi FS, Lawrence D, Lezcano C, et al. Bevacizumab plus ipilimumab in patients with metastatic melanoma. Cancer Immunol Res 2014;2(7):632–42.
51. Mellman I, Coukos G, Dranoff G. Cancer immunotherapy comes of age. Nature 2011;480(7378):480–9.

Advanced Melanoma
Resistance Mechanisms to Current Therapies

Alexandra M. Haugh, MD, MPH[a], April K.S. Salama, MD[b],
Douglas B. Johnson, MD, MSCI[c],*

KEYWORDS

- Immune checkpoint inhibitor • Immunotherapy • Resistance • BRAF inhibitor
- MEK inhibitor • Melanoma

KEY POINTS

- Novel targeted therapies and immune checkpoint inhibitors have transformed the management of advanced melanoma, although resistance limits this benefit.
- Immune checkpoint inhibitors are often associated with intrinsic resistance and primary progressive disease, which may be due to lack of immune recognition, T-cell exclusion, or alternative causes of T-cell exhaustion.
- Targeted therapies are more often associated with acquired resistance, which may in part be due to reactivation of MAP kinase signaling and transcriptomic reprogramming.

INTRODUCTION

Advances over the past decade have brought about remarkable changes in the treatment of metastatic melanoma. The introduction of targeted therapies including BRAF and MEK inhibitors as well as immune checkpoint inhibitors (ICIs) led to dramatically improved outcomes compared with chemotherapy, which had not been shown to improve survival in any large randomized trials. Although impressive outcomes are seen in some patients, responses to these agents are heterogeneous. Initial robust responses to BRAF/MEK inhibitors are complicated by eventual disease progression in most treated patients. ICIs may induce more durable long-term responses in some cases, yet a significant proportion of patients do not respond to these agents (innate resistance) or respond transiently followed by progression (acquired resistance). This review provides an overview of recent insights into innate and acquired resistance to both targeted therapies and checkpoint inhibition in metastatic melanoma. Further

[a] Department of Medicine, Vanderbilt University Medical Center, 719 Thompson Lane, Suite 20400, Nashville, TN 37204, USA; [b] Department of Medicine, Duke University Medical Center, 20 Duke Medicine Cir, Durham, NC 27710, USA; [c] Department of Medicine, Vanderbilt University Medical Center, Vanderbilt Ingram Cancer Center, 777 PRB, 2220 Pierce Avenue, Nashville, TN 37232, USA
* Corresponding author.
E-mail address: douglas.b.johnson@vumc.org

Hematol Oncol Clin N Am 35 (2021) 111–128
https://doi.org/10.1016/j.hoc.2020.09.005
0889-8588/21/© 2020 Elsevier Inc. All rights reserved.

hemonc.theclinics.com

understanding of the mechanisms involved in resistance is warranted to inform optimal clinical decision making in individual patients as well as to drive therapeutic advances that continue to improve outcomes.

DISCUSSION
Resistance to Checkpoint Inhibitors

Mutational and neoantigen burden

Several studies have demonstrated a correlation between higher tumor mutational burden and response to checkpoint inhibition with either anti-PD-1/PD-L1 or anti-CTLA-4.[1-7] Malignant cells are often detected by immune surveillance through recognition of tumor-derived neoantigens that are foreign and thus immunogenic.[8] As these neoantigens are a result of somatic mutations, higher mutational load is thought to contribute to a wider and more robust spectrum of neoantigens that can be recognized by the immune system. Tumors deficient in mismatch repair, regardless of tissue of origin, are also particularly sensitive to immune checkpoint inhibition.[9-11] These tumors are characterized by a very high frequency of somatic alterations, with a mutational load 10 to 100-fold greater than those that are mismatch-proficient, which likely plays a role in response to ICI.[12]

Recognition of a specific neoantigen may be complicated by the spectrum of different mutations within clusters of malignant cells in each tumor. Clonal neoantigen burden has been associated with response to ICI while a high burden of sub-clonal alterations was seen in tumors that progressed on therapy.[13,14] Cytotoxic chemotherapy may potentiate production of sub-clonal neoantigens, possibly contributing to decreased efficacy of ICI in some patients despite an overall high mutational burden.[14] Neoantigens that arise earlier in tumorigenesis and are shared by most cancer cells are likely to trigger a more robust immune response.

Most melanoma tumors are driven by UV-induced mutagenesis with a high frequency of somatic mutations. Subtypes of melanoma that are less likely to be UV-mediated, such as mucosal or acral melanoma, tend to have fewer point mutations but more frequent somatic structural or copy number aberrations.[15] Given the lower overall mutational burden and likely decreased neoantigen production, it is speculated that these subtypes may be less likely to respond to ICIs. Indeed, several studies report lower response rates in these noncutaneous melanomas.[16-18] Conversely, desmoplastic melanomas, which have the highest mutational burdens of all melanomas, also have the highest response rates.[19] Miao and colleagues[13] stratified melanoma tumors based on mutational signature, which included UV-associated, those associated with exposure to alkylating agents and tumors not clearly associated with specific environmental exposures. When stratified based on dominant mutational signature, there was no significant difference in mutational burden between patients with progressive disease and those who responded to immunotherapy.[13] The authors thus postulated that mutational burden may actually serve as a marker of underlying pathobiology that promotes immunogenicity rather than a true mechanism of response to therapy in melanoma. In addition, most studies have suggested threshold effects rather than a linear relationship between response and TMB within individual tumor types.

Tumors can demonstrate selective loss of neoantigens recognized by T cells as a mechanism to avoid immune detection.[20,21] Malignant cells that express these neoantigens are selectively lost from the overall tumor population through the loss of mutant alleles or epigenetic silencing of implicated genes.[20] Neoantigens lost by tumor cells following ICI were noted to have higher affinity for MHC variants and result in stronger

TCR responses in peripheral lymphocytes than those that were retained.[22] The loss of T-cell recognized neoantigens correlates with the development of neoantigen specific reactivity amongst tumor-infiltrating lymphocytes, suggesting that T cells likely play a role in modulating immunoediting.[20]

PD-L1 expression

PD-L1 expression in tumor cells or tumor-infiltrating immune cells has unsurprisingly been correlated with response to PD-1/PD-L1 blockade in melanoma.[23–26] PD-L1 negativity, however, is not a definitive marker of resistance and studies have consistently demonstrated durable responses in some patients with PD-L1 negative tumors.[24,25,27] PD-L1 status is used to identify patients appropriate for treatment with immunotherapy in some malignancies but is of uncertain utility in melanoma, which is also associated with relatively high rates of PD-L1 positivity.[28] PD-L1 expression is frequently heterogenous over time, within individual patients or even within the same tumor. Further, several different IHC stains and cut-off values were employed in early trials, further complicating assessment of PD-L1 status.[28] Expression of PD-1 and PD-L1 are also known to be dynamic and influenced by several complex and inter-related factors within the tumor microenvironment, including interferon (IFN) or other cytokine signaling, genomic alterations or changes induced by radiation or targeted therapy.[12,29]

Specific genomic alterations

Tumors that are subject to immune surveillance may become enriched for a wide range of genomic alterations that aid in immune escape. Alterations in the gene encoding β-2-microglobulin (B2M), the invariant chain of MHC, have been shown to play a role in both innate and acquired resistance to checkpoint inhibition.[30–32] Decreased expression of MHC, whether brought about by genomic changes or other mechanisms, has been associated with lack of response to anti-PD1 (MHC-II) and anti-CTLA-4 (MHC-1).[33] Germline differences in HLA genotype may impact response to checkpoint inhibition, potentially due to a decreased spectrum of neoantigens presented by tumors with homozygous HLA alleles.[34]

Loss of function mutations in *JAK1/JAK2* have been associated with both innate and acquired resistance to PD-1/PD-L1 inhibitors in melanoma.[32,35] Tumors with *JAK1/JAK2* mutations demonstrate a lack of response to IFN-γ stimulation, including a lack of associated PD-L1 expression.[32,35] Several genomic defects in the IFN-γ pathway have also been identified amongst tumors that do not respond to CTLA-4 blockade.[36] Overall these mutations appear uncommon, and likely only explain a minor proportion of resistance.

Certain tumor signaling pathways have also been shown to suppress the recruitment and diversification of T cells within the tumor microenvironment.[37,38] Activation of the WNT/β-catenin pathway in melanoma contributed to T-cell exclusion in mouse models, evidenced by a complete lack of T-cell infiltrate in many tumors.[37] Single cell RNA sampling of melanoma tumor cells treated with ICI identified a specific transcription factor, TCF7, that served as a marker of response regardless of the extent of lymphocytic invasion. This transcription factor plays a role in the Wnt/β-catenin signaling pathway and is involved with cytotoxic T-cell auto-renewal, differentiation and persistence.[39] The loss of PTEN within tumor cells has been correlated with decreased T-cell infiltration, increased expression of immunosuppressive cytokines and overall inferior clinical response to ICI.[40,41]

Recent evidence has suggested that the MAPK pathway may play a role in immune escape through upregulation of VEGF and other immunosuppressive cytokines in addition to other unknown mechanisms.[42,43] BRAF inhibitors have been shown to increase intratumoral T-cell infiltration and result in a more favorable TME with fewer immunosuppressive cytokines, fewer myeloid-derived suppressor stem cells and decreased PD-L1 expression, whereas other studies have suggested a low CD8+ T-cell infiltrate at the time of progression on BRAF inhibitors.[44–48] Acquired resistance to BRAF inhibition has been associated with upregulation of PD-L1 on tumor cells and treatment with MAPK inhibitors can induce transcriptional signatures similar to the IPRES signature associated with ICI resistance.[47,49] It remains unclear if and how changes induced by BRAF inhibition impact subsequent response to ICI in melanoma yet molecular evidence is suggestive of overlapping resistance mechanisms to both classes of therapy.[50,51] Retrospective analysis found higher response rates to first-line immunotherapy among *NRAS*-mutant melanoma compared with *BRAF* or *BRAF/NRAS* wild-type melanoma although these data have not been validated extensively.[52] The impact of MAPK pathway alterations in the development of ICI resistance is yet to be defined.

Tumor microenvironment

Malignant cells use a variety of mechanisms to evade immune destruction, many of which involve alterations in the surrounding tumor microenvironment that create an immunosuppressive barrier. The presence of tumor-infiltrating lymphocytes within the TME is associated with improved outcomes across wide spectrum of malignancies.[53] Higher numbers of intratumoral CD8+ T cells, both in the core and at the invasive margin, are predictive of response to anti-PD-1 therapy in melanoma, particularly if they express PD-1.[27,54] Functional analysis of TILs that expressed high amounts of both PD-1 and CTLA-4 revealed a partially exhausted CD8+ T-cell phenotype that could be restored to a fully activated state on PD-1/PD-L1 inhibition.[27]

Persistent antigen exposure and activation is complicated by eventual T-cell exhaustion both in the setting of ICI therapy and natural immune surveillance. The interaction between PD-1 and PD-L1 contributes significantly to the loss of effector T-cell function exhibited by exhausted CD8+ T cells.[55] Blockade of PD-L1/PD-1 can re-invigorate exhausted cytotoxic T cells; an abundance of partially exhausted CD8+ T cells within the TME has been shown to correlate with response to ICI.[27]

These re-invigorated T cells, however, will revert back to an exhausted state in the face of continued and persistent antigen exposure and do not exhibit a memory T-cell phenotype upon antigen clearance.[56] Recent studies have uncovered a hardwired epigenetic profile unique to exhausted T cells that may limit prolonged response to checkpoint inhibition and contribute to acquired resistance.[57,58] Epigenetic therapies have been proposed as a potential mechanism to overcome T-cell exhaustion and are being evaluated as an adjunct to ICI in refractory patients in ongoing trials.

The PD-1/PD-L1 interaction drives adaptive resistance through several additional mechanisms, many of which are the result of negative feedback interactions within the TME that upregulate PD-L1 expression.[12] PD-L1 plays a role in induction and maintenance of regulatory T cells and immunosuppressive myeloid cells within the TME, which are of uncertain significance in predicting response to ICI.[59,60] CTLA-4 inhibitors have been shown to result in upregulation of CD4(+)Foxp3(−) T cells within the tumor microenvironment, which express PD-1 but lack cytotoxic function and express Treg-associated markers.[61] Treatment with both PD-1/PD-L1 and CTLA-4 antibodies notably mitigates this effect in many cases and persistence of these cells after anti-PD-1 correlates with poor prognosis.[62]

A group of 26 transcriptomic signatures, collectively referred to as the innate anti-PD-1 resistance (IPRES) signature, were found to be co-enriched in pre-treatment

ICI-resistant melanomas.[63] This signature donates upregulation of genes involved with mesenchymal transition, angiogenesis and wound healing. Epithelial to mesenchymal transition has been associated with an increased presence of various immune checkpoint molecules, regulatory T cells and immunosuppressive cytokines.[64–66] The epithelial to mesenchymal transition signature is notably associated with TNFα, which promotes phenotypic plasticity and upregulation of an innate resistance signature through translational reprogramming.[67]

Both type I and II interferon signaling play an important role in T-cell activation required for initial response to checkpoint inhibition yet prolonged IFN signaling has also been associated with immune supression.[68] Interferon signaling accordingly plays a complicated role in modulating response to checkpoint inhibition. Increased expression of IFN-γ and IFN-related genes has been associated with response to anti-PD-1 in melanoma and defects in IFN signaling pathways have been associated with acquired resistance.[32,69] Gene expression studies have also identified an interferon- γ related GEP that was necessary, but not always sufficient, for clinical benefit across tumor types exposed to ICI.[70]

Persistent IFN signaling induces epigenomic and genomic alterations within tumors that dampen immune response, including expression of PD-L1 as well as upregulation of multiple additional T-cell inhibitory receptors.[71] IFN-γ may also play a role in expediting cytotoxic T-cell–dependent immunoediting.[72] As noted above, response to anti-PD-1 has been associated with a T-cell–rich inflammatory TME, characterized by an abundance of TILs and PD-L1 expression. A responsive TME is also likely one that is, "adaptive immune resistant" and further categorization of the cellular and molecular changes associated with adaptive immunity may help inform treatment decisions or uncover new therapeutic targets.[70]

Proteomic profiling found immunotherapy-responsive tumors to be enriched for proteins involved with oxidative phosphorylation and lipid metabolism compared with non-responsive samples. These samples were also enriched for antigen presentation and IFN signaling. Functional studies demonstrated that increased lipid metabolism led to upregulation of antigen expression by melanoma cells, increasing immunogenicity and potential for ICI response.[73]

The host microbiome

Increasing evidence suggests that the intestinal microbiome plays an important role in a wide variety of inflammatory or immune-mediated conditions. Increased microbial biodiversity within the host microbiome has been associated with response to PD-1 inhibition in melanoma.[74] Specific bacterial species have also been noted to be prevalent among responders, whereas others are associated with a lack of response.[74–76] Xenografted germ-free mice transplanted with stool samples from responding patients demonstrated improved outcomes with anti-PD-1 compared with those transplanted from non-responders.[76] Concurrent and prior antibiotic therapy has also been correlated with decreased response to ICI.[77,78] High dietary fiber intake has been shown to contribute to an immunostimulatory landscape within the microbiome and patients with melanoma who self-reported a high-fiber diet were significantly more likely to respond to anti-PD-1 agents.[79,80]

Overcoming immune checkpoint inhibitors resistance

Several strategies have been proposed to augment cytotoxic T-cell priming and tumor infiltration integral to ICI response, which were in part mentioned above. The full spectrum of current combination therapy approaches are beyond the scope of this review. Radiation therapy broadens the spectrum of T-cell-receptors among tumor-infiltrating lymphocytes, which may help to overcome innate or acquired mechanisms of resistance involving T-cell exclusion.[81] Melanoma vaccines may also augment the effect of checkpoint inhibition, particularly when directed toward particular neoantigens associated with a robust response to ICI.[7,82] The combination of checkpoint inhibitors and cancer vaccines, including individualized vaccines directed at neoantigens shown to demonstrate immunogenicity within a specific tumor, are currently under investigation in early phase trials.[82]

Certain oncolytic viruses capitalize on defective interferon signaling to enter and replicate within cells and may therefore be used to target IFN- γ deficient clones and overcome associated resistance.[83] Agonists of the stimulator for interferon genes (STING) receptor may increase sensitivity to checkpoint inhibition by increasing PD-L1 expression through upregulation of the JAK/STAT pathway.[84,85] A resistance program associated with T-cell exclusion and immune evasion identified by single cell RNA sequencing was also found to be repressed by CDK4/6 inhibition when given in combination with ICI in mouse models.[86] Other approaches, including co-stimulation of additional immune checkpoints, toll-like receptor agonists, and tumor-infiltrating lymphocytes may also have promise. Antibodies targeting the T-cell inhibitory receptor lymphocyte activation gene-3 (LAG-3) showed promise when used with nivolumab in melanoma refractory to anti-PD-1/PD-L1 and are being evaluated with anti-CTLA-4 in this setting as well as with anti-PD-1/PD-L1 in ICI-naïve patients (NCT03978611, NCT03743766).[87] Engagement of toll-like receptors within the TME promotes innate immune activation and associated proinflammatory cytokine production that can increase intratumoral T-cell infiltration and potentiate response to ICI.[88] Early phase trials have shown encouraging results in anti-PD-1/PDL-1 refractory patients treated with an intratumoral TLR9 agonist and ipilimumab with an overall response rate of 47% (7 of 15 patients).[89] Adoptive cell therapy with autologous tumor-infiltrating lymphocytes has been attempted and refined in melanoma for several decades with more recent trials limited to those who have progressed on standard therapies. TIL therapy optimized with pre-infusion lymphodepletion and a post-transfer IL-2 regimen resulted in durable response in some refractory patients with an ORR of 36.4% and a median duration of response that was not reached after 17 months.[90]

Resistance to BRAF/MEK Inhibitors

Mutations in *BRAF* occur in almost half of all melanomas and thus represent a major therapeutic target. A majority of *BRAF*-mutant melanomas harbor a substitution at codon 600 of the *BRAF* gene, which results in constitutive kinase activation and downstream activation of the MAPK pathway. The MAPK pathway plays a role in a wide spectrum of intracellular processes, including differentiation, stress response, and cell survival, which it also regulates via physiologic negative feedback mechanisms. Constitutive activation of the MAPK pathway results in unregulated cell growth and proliferation that drives tumorigenesis.

The development of small molecule inhibitors specific to the *BRAF*-mutant kinase (BRAFi) represented a major breakthrough in the treatment of melanoma. These agents were associated with significantly improved overall response rates, progression-free survival (PFS) and overall survival (OS) when compared with chemotherapy in patients with *BRAF* V600 mutant melanoma.[91,92] Primary resistance to BRAF inhibition is relatively rare, with impressive initial response in many patients, yet these regimens are frequently complicated by acquired resistance. Unlike many other malignancies treated with other targeted kinase inhibitors, which often develop resistance through "gate-keeper" mutations that impede interaction between the inhibitor and the mutated kinase, *BRAF*-mutated melanomas use several complex alternative mechanisms to upregulate the downstream MAPK pathway and bring about resistance.

Evidence that re-activation of the MAPK pathway was involved with acquired resistance to BRAFi led to the introduction of combined therapy with both BRAF and MEK inhibition (MEKi). MEK is directly downstream from BRAF in the MAPK cascade and MEKi was independently associated with superior outcomes compared with chemotherapy in patients with *BRAF* V600 mutant melanoma.[93] Targeting multiple sites along the MAPK pathway with the addition of MEKi was proposed in an attempt to mitigate eventual resistance as well as to promote a more robust response to therapy. Multiple trials demonstrated significant improvement in response rate, PFS and OS with both BRAF and MEK inhibitors compared with BRAFi monotherapy and combination therapy became standard of care in *BRAF* V600 mutant melanoma.[94–96]

Despite significant improvements with combination therapy, BRAF/MEK inhibition is still frequently complicated by eventual resistance, most often via upregulation of MAPK signaling. Although many studies have focused on categorizing BRAF inhibitor resistance in melanoma, resistance to the BRAF/MEKi combination is due to similar mechanisms.[97–99] Eventual resistance to BRAF/MEKi should be expected in most patients, yet recently published follow-up data from the COMBI-v and COMBI-d trials suggests the potential for long-term benefit in a minority of patients treated with BRAF + MEK inhibitiors.[100] Patients who demonstrated a complete response to therapy (109 of 563%, 19%) had a 5-year OS of 71% compared with 34% in the overall cohort. Several baseline factors were also found to be associated with prolonged PFS including older age, female sex, normal lactate dehydrogenase level, and less than three organ sites with distant metastasis. Patients who demonstrated a complete response shared similar baseline factors. PFS at 5 years was observed in approximately 15% of the population.[100] Longer-term follow-up of patients with sustained response to BRAF/MEKi as well as further molecular and clinical characterization of this sub-group is warranted.

The categorization of BRAF/MEKi resistance is complicated by a diverse array of mechanisms with significant heterogeneity between patients and within individual tumors. While a single predominant resistance mechanism may be identified in one resistant tumor sample, additional biopsies from the same patient often demonstrate distinct or unknown drivers of resistance.[99] Melanoma clones emerging after BRAFi therapy demonstrate branched evolution and some tumors can proliferate in the setting of BRAFi in the absence of any clear genomic driver.[101] Intra-tumor heterogeneity can be explained in part by a suspected multi-step pattern of resistance acquisition. This starts with adaptive transcriptional reprogramming that allows for cell survival in the presence of BRAFi via phenotypic plasticity as well as increased signaling in alternative RTK pathways that frequently converge with the MAPK pathway. This adaptive transcriptional state allows tumor cells to survive long enough to acquire "fixed" mediators of resistance, which are often genomically mediated.

Increasing evidence suggests melanoma cells exposed to BRAF inhibition may capitalize on an innate stress reaction that promotes transition to a "slow-growth" phenotypic state associated with oncogene-induced senescence and de-differentiation as well as changes in chromatin remodeling and histone deacetylase activity.[102–104] Transcriptomic analysis of BRAF/MEKi resistant tumors demonstrated recurrent involvement of specific genes and pathways, which frequently demonstrated differential methylation of tumor cell-intrinsic CpG sites.[105]

The early adaptive "persister" state adopted by some melanoma cells in response to BRAF inhibition has also been associated with phenotypic transition to a more de-differentiated mesenchymal state.[106,107] Overexpression of the transcription factor c-JUN has been associated with a mesenchymal gene signature and an EMT-like phenotypic transition signature in melanoma cells.[108,109] Inhibition of c-JUN, either via direct silencing or upstream inhibition of c-JUN amino-terminal kinase (JNK), has been shown to increase overall cell death and decrease the population of "persister" cells when used in combination with BRAF inhibitors.[106,108,109] Microphthalmia associated transcription factor (MITF), a transcription factor that controls multiple genes integral to melanocyte function, has been repeatedly implicated in BRAF/MEK inhibitor resistance. While some studies have implicated MITF upregulation as a mechanism of BRAF resistance, a majority have demonstrated the emergence of "MITF-low" populations early in the course of acquired resistance.[110–113]

In addition to re-activation of MAPK signaling, increased signaling in the PI3 kinase/AKT pathway has also been implicated in de novo and acquired resistance to BRAF/MEK inhibition in almost 20% of melanoma patients.[114] MAPK pathway inhibition has been shown to induce upregulation of AKT signaling in resistant cells and high levels of AKT activity have been correlated with a lack of response to MEK inhibition in patients with *BRAF*-mutant melanoma.[114–116] Despite encouraging pre-clinical data, inhibitors of PI3K or downstream PI3K pathway effector molecules have largely failed to offer additional clinical benefit when used in combination with BRAF/MEK inhibitors in early stage trials.[117]

Increased signaling in the MAPK and PI3K pathways in resistant cells is modulated by multiple additional RTK pathways that are frequently upregulated in the setting of BRAF/MEKi resistance.[118–123] Evidence suggests that treatment with BRAFi more likely results in the coordinated upregulation of multiple RTKs in individual tumor cells rather than selective upregulation of specific receptors that may be amenable to therapeutic intervention.[117] Additional RTK pathways shown to be upregulated in resistant cells include epidermal growth factor receptor (EGFR), ERBB3, hepatocyte growth factor receptor (c-MET), platelet derived growth factor (PDGFR)-a, and the insulin like growth factor (IGF)-1 receptor.[118–123] Some studies have demonstrated an inverse correlation between MITF expression in resistant samples and upregulation of multiple RTKs, including the RTK AXL, which is over-expressed in many advanced malignancies and often associated with acquired resistance to chemotherapy.[110–112,124]

Melanoma cells capable of adapting to MAPK inhibition will eventually acquire permanent genomic alterations that confer resistance to therapy. Genomic profiling studies have demonstrated a wide spectrum of genetic drivers associated with MAPKi resistance with significant intrapatient and intratumoral heterogeneity. As expected, most identified mutations are associated with increased signaling within the MAPK pathway, which is restored in an estimated 80% of patients resistant to dabrafenib or vemurafenib.[125] These include activating mutations in NRAS and/or MEK1/2 as well as *BRAF* V600 amplifications and *BRAF* splice site variants.[99,118,126] Non-MAPK pathway alterations most frequently involve increased signaling through the PI3K pathway.[99,101,127] Copy number variations in CDKN2A and CCND1 and inactivation of Rb have also been implicated in decreased response to BRAF/MEK inhibition although it is unclear whether this is due to more aggressive disease overall or a specific mechanistic link to resistance.[128,129]

Overcoming BRAF/MEK inhibitor resistance

Given the role of persistent MAPK signaling in resistance to BRAF/MEKi, inhibition farther downstream in the pathway was proposed as a potential mechanism to mitigate MAPK re-activation. Mitogen-activated extracellular-signal regulated kinase (ERK) is the final effector in the MAPK cascade and acts within the nucleus to promote proliferation, growth and survival. Pre-clinical studies have suggested that ERK inhibitors can independently induce regression in *BRAF*-mutant melanoma and may also reverse resistance to BRAF/MEKi.[130] ERK inhibitors have produced responses in BRAF/MEKi resistant patients as well as treatment naïve *BRAF* and *NRAS*-mutant melanomas in small early clinical trials.[131,132]

Re-introduction of BRAF/MEKi in patients who previously progressed on these agents has notably led to significant responses in some cases.[133] Intermittent dosing of BRAFi has also induced more durable responses in mouse models compared with continuous dosing with regression of BRAF-amplified resistant tumors following BRAFi discontinuation.[114,134] Evidence suggests that some BRAF/MEKi resistant melanomas may become "inhibitor addicted" and regress with short-term drug withdrawal.[135] Intermittent dosing strategies may improve outcomes in these patients and are being evaluated in early phase trials (NCT02196181). However, one study recently presented negative results with a regimen of 5 weeks on and 3 weeks off dabrafenib and trametinib compared with continuous dosing.[136]

The AXL receptor is a target of interest in many malignancies, particularly in the setting of refractory or advanced disease.[137] Several therapeutic agents are under investigation in early trials, including established multi-targeted kinase inhibitors shown to inhibit AXL and novel more specific small molecule inhibitors.[138,139] AXL-directed antibody-drug-conjugates (ADC) have also been developed in an attempt to more specifically target AXL-expressing cell populations. When used in combination with BRAF/MEKi in patient-derived xenografts of melanoma with heterogeneous cell populations, an ADC containing the antimitotic agent monomethyl auristatin E (AXL-107-MMAE) eliminated tumor cells in the AXL-high population while BRAF/MEKi were effective in AXL-low cell lines. AXL-107-MMAE was also shown to potentiate the effect of BRAF/MEKi in AXL-low populations by exploiting BRAF/MEKi-induced transcriptional upregulation of AXL, suggesting a potential for benefit in BRAF/MEKi naïve patients. A phase I trial evaluating an AXL-specific ADC in advanced or relapsed/refractory solid tumors is ongoing (NCT02988817).

Inhibitors of heat shock protein-90 (HSP90), a chaperone that supports many RTKs and intracellular proteins involved in tumor growth and progression, have also been suggested as an adjunct therapy that may mitigate BRAF/MEKi resistance in melanoma. A phase trial I evaluating the HSP90 inhibitor XL888 and vemurafenib in BRAFi naïve patients with *BRAF*-mutant melanoma demonstrated a notable 75% response rate (15 of 20 evaluable patients) in addition to a tolerable toxicity profile.[140] Multiple phase I trials are evaluating the use of these agents with dual BRAF/MEKi (NCT02721459, NCT02097225).

SUMMARY

Despite the recent advances in melanoma treatment, resistance to currently available immune and targeted therapies remains the major barriers to long-term disease control in many patients. Most often, this is associated with intrinsic/innate resistance to ICIs and acquired resistance to BRAF and MEK kinase inhibitors. Mechanisms of resistance are diverse and will require innovative and perhaps personalized management strategies.

CLINICS CARE POINTS

- Although resistance to BRAF and MEK inhibitors is a major clinical problem, patients have high response rates to BRAF and MEK inhibitor retreatment after at least 6 weeks off therapy.
- Patients with melanoma progressing on anti-PD-1 (with either acquired or intrinsic resistance) may benefit from adding ipilimumab to their anti-PD-1 therapy, with response rates of 25-30%.

DISCLOSURE

Dr A.K.S. Salama receives research funding (paid to institution) from Bristol Myers Squibb, Immunocore, Merck and has served as a consultant/advisory board member for Array, Novartis, Iovance and Regeneron. Dr D.B. Johnson serves on advisory boards for Array Biopharma, BMS, Iovance, Jansen, Merck, and Novartis, and receives research funding from BMS and Incyte.

REFERENCES

1. Yarchoan M, Hopkins A, Jaffee EM. Tumor mutational burden and response rate to PD-1 inhibition. N Engl J Med 2017;377(25):2500–1.
2. Samstein RM, Lee CH, Shoushtari AN, et al. Tumor mutational load predicts survival after immunotherapy across multiple cancer types. Nat Genet 2019;51(2): 202–6.
3. Johnson DB, Frampton GM, Rioth MJ, et al. Targeted next generation sequencing identifies markers of response to PD-1 blockade. Cancer Immunol Res 2016;4(11):959–67.
4. Van Allen EM, Miao D, Schilling B, et al. Genomic correlates of response to CTLA-4 blockade in metastatic melanoma. Science 2015;350(6257):207–11.
5. Rizvi NA, Hellmann MD, Snyder A, et al. Cancer immunology. Mutational landscape determines sensitivity to PD-1 blockade in non-small cell lung cancer. Science 2015;348(6230):124–8.
6. Hellmann MD, Ciuleanu TE, Pluzanski A, et al. Nivolumab plus Ipilimumab in Lung Cancer with a High Tumor Mutational Burden. N Engl J Med 2018; 378(22):2093–104.
7. Snyder A, Makarov V, Merghoub T, et al. Genetic basis for clinical response to CTLA-4 blockade in melanoma. N Engl J Med 2014;371(23):2189–99.
8. van Rooij N, van Buuren MM, Philips D, et al. Tumor exome analysis reveals neoantigen-specific T-cell reactivity in an ipilimumab-responsive melanoma. J Clin Oncol 2013;31(32):e439–42.
9. Le DT, Durham JN, Smith KN, et al. Mismatch repair deficiency predicts response of solid tumors to PD-1 blockade. Science 2017;357(6349):409–13.
10. Lipson EJ, Sharfman WH, Drake CG, et al. Durable cancer regression off-treatment and effective reinduction therapy with an anti-PD-1 antibody. Clin Cancer Res 2013;19(2):462–8.
11. Le DT, Uram JN, Wang H, et al. PD-1 blockade in tumors with mismatch-repair deficiency. N Engl J Med 2015;372(26):2509–20.
12. You W, Shang B, Sun J, et al. Mechanistic insight of predictive biomarkers for antitumor PD-1/PD-L1 blockade: A paradigm shift towards immunome evaluation (Review). Oncol Rep 2020;44(2):424–37.

13. Miao D, Margolis CA, Vokes NI, et al. Genomic correlates of response to immune checkpoint blockade in microsatellite-stable solid tumors. Nat Genet 2018; 50(9):1271–81.
14. McGranahan N, Furness AJ, Rosenthal R, et al. Clonal neoantigens elicit T cell immunoreactivity and sensitivity to immune checkpoint blockade. Science 2016; 351(6280):1463–9.
15. Hayward NK, Wilmott JS, Waddell N, et al. Whole-genome landscapes of major melanoma subtypes. Nature 2017;545(7653):175–80.
16. Shoushtari AN, Munhoz RR, Kuk D, et al. The efficacy of anti-PD-1 agents in acral and mucosal melanoma. Cancer 2016;122(21):3354–62.
17. Johnson DB, Peng C, Abramson RG, et al. Clinical Activity of Ipilimumab in Acral Melanoma: A Retrospective Review. Oncologist 2015;20(6):648–52.
18. Nakamura Y, Namikawa K, Yoshino K, et al. Anti-PD1 checkpoint inhibitor therapy in acral melanoma: a multicenter study of 193 Japanese patients. Ann Oncol 2020;31(9):1198–206.
19. Eroglu Z, Zaretsky JM, Hu-Lieskovan S, et al. High response rate to PD-1 blockade in desmoplastic melanomas. Nature 2018;553(7688):347–50.
20. Verdegaal EM, de Miranda NF, Visser M, et al. Neoantigen landscape dynamics during human melanoma-T cell interactions. Nature 2016;536(7614):91–5.
21. Matsushita H, Vesely MD, Koboldt DC, et al. Cancer exome analysis reveals a T-cell-dependent mechanism of cancer immunoediting. Nature 2012; 482(7385):400–4.
22. Anagnostou V, Smith KN, Forde PM, et al. Evolution of neoantigen landscape during immune checkpoint blockade in non-small cell lung cancer. Cancer Discov 2017;7(3):264–76.
23. Topalian SL, Hodi FS, Brahmer JR, et al. Safety, activity, and immune correlates of anti-PD-1 antibody in cancer. N Engl J Med 2012;366(26):2443–54.
24. Weber JS, Kudchadkar RR, Yu B, et al. Safety, efficacy, and biomarkers of nivolumab with vaccine in ipilimumab-refractory or -naive melanoma. J Clin Oncol 2013;31(34):4311–8.
25. Larkin J, Chiarion-Sileni V, Gonzalez R, et al. Combined nivolumab and ipilimumab or monotherapy in untreated melanoma. N Engl J Med 2015;373(1):23–34.
26. Robert C, Long GV, Brady B, et al. Nivolumab in previously untreated melanoma without BRAF mutation. N Engl J Med 2015;372(4):320–30.
27. Daud AI, Loo K, Pauli ML, et al. Tumor immune profiling predicts response to anti-PD-1 therapy in human melanoma. J Clin Invest 2016;126(9):3447–52.
28. Taube JM, Klein A, Brahmer JR, et al. Association of PD-1, PD-1 ligands, and other features of the tumor immune microenvironment with response to anti-PD-1 therapy. Clin Cancer Res 2014;20(19):5064–74.
29. Bald T, Landsberg J, Lopez-Ramos D, et al. Immune cell-poor melanomas benefit from PD-1 blockade after targeted type I IFN activation. Cancer Discov 2014;4(6):674–87.
30. Rooney MS, Shukla SA, Wu CJ, et al. Molecular and genetic properties of tumors associated with local immune cytolytic activity. Cell 2015;160(1–2):48–61.
31. Zhao F, Sucker A, Horn S, et al. Melanoma lesions independently acquire T-cell resistance during metastatic latency. Cancer Res 2016;76(15):4347–58.
32. Zaretsky JM, Garcia-Diaz A, Shin DS, et al. Mutations associated with acquired resistance to PD-1 blockade in melanoma. N Engl J Med 2016;375(9):819–29.
33. Rodig SJ, Gusenleitner D, Jackson DG, et al. MHC proteins confer differential sensitivity to CTLA-4 and PD-1 blockade in untreated metastatic melanoma. Sci Transl Med 2018;10(450):eaar3342.

34. Chowell D, Morris LGT, Grigg CM, et al. Patient HLA class I genotype influences cancer response to checkpoint blockade immunotherapy. Science 2018; 359(6375):582–7.

35. Shin DS, Zaretsky JM, Escuin-Ordinas H, et al. Primary resistance to PD-1 blockade mediated by JAK1/2 mutations. Cancer Discov 2017;7(2):188–201.

36. Gao J, Shi LZ, Zhao H, et al. Loss of IFN-γ pathway genes in tumor cells as a mechanism of Resistance to Anti-CTLA-4 Therapy. Cell 2016;167(2): 397–404.e9.

37. Spranger S, Bao R, Gajewski TF. Melanoma-intrinsic β-catenin signalling prevents anti-tumour immunity. Nature 2015;523(7559):231–5.

38. Spranger S, Luke JJ, Bao R, et al. Density of immunogenic antigens does not explain the presence or absence of the T-cell-inflamed tumor microenvironment in melanoma. Proc Natl Acad Sci U S A 2016;113(48):E7759–68.

39. Sade-Feldman M, Yizhak K, Bjorgaard SL, et al. Defining T cell states associated with response to checkpoint immunotherapy in melanoma. Cell 2018;175(4): 998–1013.e20.

40. Peng W, Chen JQ, Liu C, et al. Loss of PTEN promotes resistance to T cell-mediated immunotherapy. Cancer Discov 2016;6(2):202–16.

41. George S, Miao D, Demetri GD, et al. Loss of PTEN is associated with resistance to anti-PD-1 checkpoint blockade therapy in metastatic uterine leiomyosarcoma. Immunity 2017;46(2):197–204.

42. Boni A, Cogdill AP, Dang P, et al. Selective BRAFV600E inhibition enhances T-cell recognition of melanoma without affecting lymphocyte function. Cancer Res 2010;70(13):5213–9.

43. Liu C, Peng W, Xu C, et al. BRAF inhibition increases tumor infiltration by T cells and enhances the antitumor activity of adoptive immunotherapy in mice. Clin Cancer Res 2013;19(2):393–403.

44. Frederick DT, Piris A, Cogdill AP, et al. BRAF inhibition is associated with enhanced melanoma antigen expression and a more favorable tumor microenvironment in patients with metastatic melanoma. Clin Cancer Res 2013;19(5): 1225–31.

45. Schilling B, Paschen A. Immunological consequences of selective BRAF inhibitors in malignant melanoma: Neutralization of myeloid-derived suppressor cells. Oncoimmunology 2013;2(8):e25218.

46. Wilmott JS, Long GV, Howle JR, et al. Selective BRAF inhibitors induce marked T-cell infiltration into human metastatic melanoma. Clin Cancer Res 2012;18(5): 1386–94.

47. Liu L, Mayes PA, Eastman S, et al. The BRAF and MEK inhibitors dabrafenib and trametinib: effects on immune function and in combination with immunomodulatory antibodies targeting PD-1, PD-L1, and CTLA-4. Clin Cancer Res 2015; 21(7):1639–51.

48. Cooper ZA, Reuben A, Spencer CN, et al. Distinct clinical patterns and immune infiltrates are observed at time of progression on targeted therapy versus immune checkpoint blockade for melanoma. Oncoimmunology 2016;5(3): e1136044.

49. Hugo W, Zaretsky JM, Sun L, et al. Genomic and transcriptomic features of response to anti-PD-1 therapy in metastatic melanoma. Cell 2017;168(3):542.

50. Yan Y, Wongchenko MJ, Robert C, et al. Genomic features of exceptional response in vemurafenib +/- cobimetinib-treated patients with BRAF (V600)-mutated metastatic melanoma. Clin Cancer Res 2019;25(11):3239–46.

51. Johnson DB, Pectasides E, Feld E, et al. Sequencing treatment in BRAFV600 mutant melanoma: anti-PD-1 before and after BRAF inhibition. J Immunother 2017;40(1):31–5.

52. Johnson DB, Lovly CM, Flavin M, et al. Impact of NRAS mutations for patients with advanced melanoma treated with immune therapies. Cancer Immunol Res 2015;3(3):288–95.

53. Fridman WH, Pagès F, Sautès-Fridman C, et al. The immune contexture in human tumours: impact on clinical outcome. Nat Rev Cancer 2012;12(4):298–306.

54. Tumeh PC, Harview CL, Yearley JH, et al. PD-1 blockade induces responses by inhibiting adaptive immune resistance. Nature 2014;515(7528):568–71.

55. Wherry EJ, Kurachi M. Molecular and cellular insights into T cell exhaustion. Nat Rev Immunol 2015;15(8):486–99.

56. Pauken KE, Sammons MA, Odorizzi PM, et al. Epigenetic stability of exhausted T cells limits durability of reinvigoration by PD-1 blockade. Science 2016; 354(6316):1160–5.

57. Sen DR, Kaminski J, Barnitz RA, et al. The epigenetic landscape of T cell exhaustion. Science 2016;354(6316):1165–9.

58. Mognol GP, Spreafico R, Wong V, et al. Exhaustion-associated regulatory regions in CD8(+) tumor-infiltrating T cells. Proc Natl Acad Sci U S A 2017; 114(13):E2776–85.

59. Francisco LM, Salinas VH, Brown KE, et al. PD-L1 regulates the development, maintenance, and function of induced regulatory T cells. J Exp Med 2009; 206(13):3015–29.

60. Ding ZC, Lu X, Yu M, et al. Immunosuppressive myeloid cells induced by chemotherapy attenuate antitumor CD4+ T-cell responses through the PD-1-PD-L1 axis. Cancer Res 2014;74(13):3441–53.

61. Avogadri F, Zappasodi R, Yang A, et al. Combination of alphavirus replicon particle-based vaccination with immunomodulatory antibodies: therapeutic activity in the B16 melanoma mouse model and immune correlates. Cancer Immunol Res 2014;2(5):448–58.

62. Zappasodi R, Budhu S, Hellmann MD, et al. Non-conventional Inhibitory CD4(+) Foxp3(-)PD-1(hi) T Cells as a Biomarker of Immune Checkpoint Blockade Activity. Cancer Cell 2018;33(6):1017–32.e7.

63. Hugo W, Zaretsky JM, Sun L, et al. Genomic and transcriptomic features of response to anti-PD-1 therapy in metastatic melanoma. Cell 2016;165(1):35–44.

64. Chen L, Gibbons DL, Goswami S, et al. Metastasis is regulated via microRNA-200/ZEB1 axis control of tumour cell PD-L1 expression and intratumoral immunosuppression. Nat Commun 2014;5:5241.

65. Chen L, Heymach JV, Qin FX, et al. The mutually regulatory loop of epithelial-mesenchymal transition and immunosuppression in cancer progression. Oncoimmunology 2015;4(5):e1002731.

66. Mak MP, Tong P, Diao L, et al. A patient-derived, pan-cancer EMT signature identifies global molecular alterations and immune target enrichment following epithelial-to-mesenchymal transition. Clin Cancer Res 2016;22(3):609–20.

67. Falletta P, Sanchez-Del-Campo L, Chauhan J, et al. Translation reprogramming is an evolutionarily conserved driver of phenotypic plasticity and therapeutic resistance in melanoma. Genes Dev 2017;31(1):18–33.

68. Minn AJ, Wherry EJ. Combination cancer therapies with immune checkpoint blockade: convergence on interferon signaling. Cell 2016;165(2):272–5.

69. Herbst RS, Soria JC, Kowanetz M, et al. Predictive correlates of response to the anti-PD-L1 antibody MPDL3280A in cancer patients. Nature 2014;515(7528): 563–7.
70. Ayers M, Lunceford J, Nebozhyn M, et al. IFN-γ-related mRNA profile predicts clinical response to PD-1 blockade. J Clin Invest 2017;127(8):2930–40.
71. Benci JL, Xu B, Qiu Y, et al. Tumor interferon signaling regulates a multigenic resistance program to immune checkpoint blockade. Cell 2016;167(6): 1540–54.e2.
72. Takeda K, Nakayama M, Hayakawa Y, et al. IFN-γ is required for cytotoxic T cell-dependent cancer genome immunoediting. Nat Commun 2017;8:14607.
73. Harel M, Ortenberg R, Varanasi SK, et al. Proteomics of melanoma response to immunotherapy reveals mitochondrial dependence. Cell 2019;179(1): 236–50.e8.
74. Gopalakrishnan V, Spencer CN, Nezi L, et al. Gut microbiome modulates response to anti-PD-1 immunotherapy in melanoma patients. Science 2018; 359(6371):97–103.
75. Chaput N, Lepage P, Coutzac C, et al. Baseline gut microbiota predicts clinical response and colitis in metastatic melanoma patients treated with ipilimumab. Ann Oncol 2017;28(6):1368–79.
76. Matson V, Fessler J, Bao R, et al. The commensal microbiome is associated with anti-PD-1 efficacy in metastatic melanoma patients. Science 2018;359(6371): 104–8.
77. Pinato DJ, Howlett S, Ottaviani D, et al. Association of prior antibiotic treatment with survival and response to immune checkpoint inhibitor therapy in patients with cancer. JAMA Oncol 2019;5(12):1774–8.
78. Routy B, Le Chatelier E, Derosa L, et al. Gut microbiome influences efficacy of PD-1-based immunotherapy against epithelial tumors. Science 2018; 359(6371):91–7.
79. Benus RF, van der Werf TS, Welling GW, et al. Association between Faecalibacterium prausnitzii and dietary fibre in colonic fermentation in healthy human subjects. Br J Nutr 2010;104(5):693–700.
80. Spencer CN, Gopalakrishnan V, McQuade JL. The gut microbiome (GM) and immunotherapy response are influenced by host lifestyle factors. American Association of Cancer Research Annual Meeting. Chicago, April 2019.
81. Twyman-Saint Victor C, Rech AJ, Maity A, et al. Radiation and dual checkpoint blockade activate non-redundant immune mechanisms in cancer. Nature 2015; 520(7547):373–7.
82. Maurer DM, Butterfield LH, Vujanovic L. Melanoma vaccines: clinical status and immune endpoints. Melanoma Res 2019;29(2):109–18.
83. Zamarin D, Holmgaard RB, Subudhi SK, et al. Localized oncolytic virotherapy overcomes systemic tumor resistance to immune checkpoint blockade immunotherapy. Sci Transl Med 2014;6(226):226ra232.
84. Fu J, Kanne DB, Leong M, et al. STING agonist formulated cancer vaccines can cure established tumors resistant to PD-1 blockade. Sci Transl Med 2015; 7(283):283ra252.
85. Fares CM, Van Allen EM, Drake CG, et al. Mechanisms of resistance to immune checkpoint blockade: why does checkpoint inhibitor immunotherapy not work for all patients? Am Soc Clin Oncol Educ Book 2019;39:147–64.
86. Jerby-Arnon L, Shah P, Cuoco MS, et al. A cancer cell program promotes t cell exclusion and resistance to checkpoint blockade. Cell 2018;175(4):984–97.e4.

87. Ascierto P, Melero I, Bhatia S et al. Initial efficacy of anti-lymphocyte activation gene-3 (anti–LAG-3; BMS-986016) in combination with nivolumab (nivo) in pts with melanoma (MEL) previously treated with anti–PD-1/PD-L1 therapy. Journal of Clinical Oncology 2017;35:9520.

88. Reilley MJ, Morrow B, Ager CR, et al. TLR9 activation cooperates with T cell checkpoint blockade to regress poorly immunogenic melanoma. J Immunother Cancer 2019;7(1):323.

89. Diab A RS, Haymaker CL. A phase 2 study to evaluate the safety and efficacy of Intratumoral (IT) injection of the TLR9 agonist IMO-2125 (IMO) in combination with ipilimumab (ipi) in PD-1 inhibitor refractory melanoma. Paper presented at: 2018 Annual ASCO Meeting. Chicago, June 1, 2018.

90. Sarnaik A, KN, Chesney JA. Long-term follow up of lifileucel (LN-144) cryopreserved autologous tumor-infiltrating lymphocyte therapy in patients with advanced melanoma progressed on multiple prior therapies. Journal of Clinical Oncology 2020;38(15suppl):10006-10006.

91. Chapman PB, Robert C, Larkin J, et al. Vemurafenib in patients with BRAFV600 mutation-positive metastatic melanoma: final overall survival results of the randomized BRIM-3 study. Ann Oncol 2017;28(10):2581–7.

92. Hauschild A, Grob JJ, Demidov LV, et al. An update on BREAK-3, a phase III, randomized trial: Dabrafenib (DAB) versus dacarbazine (DTIC) in patients with BRAF V600E-positive mutation metastatic melanoma (MM). J Clin Oncol 2013;31(15_suppl):9013.

93. Flaherty KT, Robert C, Hersey P, et al. Improved survival with MEK inhibition in BRAF-mutated melanoma. N Engl J Med 2012;367(2):107–14.

94. Dummer R, Ascierto PA, Gogas HJ, et al. Overall survival in patients with BRAF-mutant melanoma receiving encorafenib plus binimetinib versus vemurafenib or encorafenib (COLUMBUS): a multicentre, open-label, randomised, phase 3 trial. Lancet Oncol 2018;19(10):1315–27.

95. Ascierto PA, McArthur GA, Dreno B, et al. Cobimetinib combined with vemurafenib in advanced BRAF(V600)-mutant melanoma (coBRIM): updated efficacy results from a randomised, double-blind, phase 3 trial. Lancet Oncol 2016; 17(9):1248–60.

96. Larkin J, Ascierto PA, Dreno B, et al. Combined vemurafenib and cobimetinib in BRAF-mutated melanoma. N Engl J Med 2014;371(20):1867–76.

97. Wagle N, Van Allen EM, Treacy DJ, et al. MAP kinase pathway alterations in BRAF-mutant melanoma patients with acquired resistance to combined RAF/MEK inhibition. Cancer Discov 2014;4(1):61–8.

98. Long GV, Fung C, Menzies AM, et al. Increased MAPK reactivation in early resistance to dabrafenib/trametinib combination therapy of BRAF-mutant metastatic melanoma. Nat Commun 2014;5:5694.

99. Johnson DB, Menzies AM, Zimmer L, et al. Acquired BRAF inhibitor resistance: A multicenter meta-analysis of the spectrum and frequencies, clinical behaviour, and phenotypic associations of resistance mechanisms. Eur J Cancer 2015; 51(18):2792–9.

100. Robert C, Grob JJ, Stroyakovskiy D, et al. Five-year outcomes with dabrafenib plus trametinib in metastatic melanoma. N Engl J Med 2019;381(7):626–36.

101. Shi H, Hugo W, Kong X, et al. Acquired resistance and clonal evolution in melanoma during BRAF inhibitor therapy. Cancer Discov 2014;4(1):80–93.

102. Ravindran Menon D, Das S, Krepler C, et al. A stress-induced early innate response causes multidrug tolerance in melanoma. Oncogene 2015;34(34):4448–59.

103. Webster MR, Xu M, Kinzler KA, et al. Wnt5A promotes an adaptive, senescent-like stress response, while continuing to drive invasion in melanoma cells. Pigment Cell Melanoma Res 2015;28(2):184–95.
104. Sun C, Wang L, Huang S, et al. Reversible and adaptive resistance to BRAF(V600E) inhibition in melanoma. Nature 2014;508(7494):118–22.
105. Hugo W, Shi H, Sun L, et al. Non-genomic and Immune Evolution of Melanoma Acquiring MAPKi Resistance. Cell 2015;162(6):1271–85.
106. Titz B, Lomova A, Le A, et al. JUN dependency in distinct early and late BRAF inhibition adaptation states of melanoma. Cell Discov 2016;2:16028.
107. Fedorenko IV, Abel EV, Koomen JM, et al. Fibronectin induction abrogates the BRAF inhibitor response of BRAF V600E/PTEN-null melanoma cells. Oncogene 2016;35(10):1225–35.
108. Ramsdale R, Jorissen RN, Li FZ, et al. The transcription cofactor c-JUN mediates phenotype switching and BRAF inhibitor resistance in melanoma. Sci Signal 2015;8(390):ra82.
109. Fallahi-Sichani M, Moerke NJ, Niepel M, et al. Systematic analysis of BRAF(V600E) melanomas reveals a role for JNK/c-Jun pathway in adaptive resistance to drug-induced apoptosis. Mol Syst Biol 2015;11(3):797.
110. Konieczkowski DJ, Johannessen CM, Abudayyeh O, et al. A melanoma cell state distinction influences sensitivity to MAPK pathway inhibitors. Cancer Discov 2014;4(7):816–27.
111. Müller J, Krijgsman O, Tsoi J, et al. Low MITF/AXL ratio predicts early resistance to multiple targeted drugs in melanoma. Nat Commun 2014;5:5712.
112. Johannessen CM, Johnson LA, Piccioni F, et al. A melanocyte lineage program confers resistance to MAP kinase pathway inhibition. Nature 2013;504(7478): 138–42.
113. Wellbrock C, Arozarena I. Microphthalmia-associated transcription factor in melanoma development and MAP-kinase pathway targeted therapy. Pigment Cell Melanoma Res 2015;28(4):390–406.
114. Lim SY, Menzies AM, Rizos H. Mechanisms and strategies to overcome resistance to molecularly targeted therapy for melanoma. Cancer 2017;123(S11): 2118–29.
115. Catalanotti F, Solit DB, Pulitzer MP, et al. Phase II trial of MEK inhibitor selumetinib (AZD6244, ARRY-142886) in patients with BRAFV600E/K-mutated melanoma. Clin Cancer Res 2013;19(8):2257–64.
116. Gopal YN, Deng W, Woodman SE, et al. Basal and treatment-induced activation of AKT mediates resistance to cell death by AZD6244 (ARRY-142886) in Braf-mutant human cutaneous melanoma cells. Cancer Res 2010;70(21):8736–47.
117. Ascierto PA, Flaherty K, Goff S. Emerging strategies in systemic therapy for the treatment of melanoma. Am Soc Clin Oncol Educ Book 2018;38:751–8.
118. Villanueva J, Vultur A, Lee JT, et al. Acquired resistance to BRAF inhibitors mediated by a RAF kinase switch in melanoma can be overcome by cotargeting MEK and IGF-1R/PI3K. Cancer Cell 2010;18(6):683–95.
119. Abel EV, Basile KJ, Kugel CH 3rd, et al. Melanoma adapts to RAF/MEK inhibitors through FOXD3-mediated upregulation of ERBB3. J Clin Invest 2013;123(5): 2155–68.
120. Nazarian R, Shi H, Wang Q, et al. Melanomas acquire resistance to B-RAF(V600E) inhibition by RTK or N-RAS upregulation. Nature 2010; 468(7326):973–7.

121. Girotti MR, Pedersen M, Sanchez-Laorden B, et al. Inhibiting EGF receptor or SRC family kinase signaling overcomes BRAF inhibitor resistance in melanoma. Cancer Discov 2013;3(2):158–67.
122. Paraiso KH, Fedorenko IV, Cantini LP, et al. Recovery of phospho-ERK activity allows melanoma cells to escape from BRAF inhibitor therapy. Br J Cancer 2010;102(12):1724–30.
123. Straussman R, Morikawa T, Shee K, et al. Tumour micro-environment elicits innate resistance to RAF inhibitors through HGF secretion. Nature 2012; 487(7408):500–4.
124. Sensi M, Catani M, Castellano G, et al. Human cutaneous melanomas lacking MITF and melanocyte differentiation antigens express a functional Axl receptor kinase. J Invest Dermatol 2011;131(12):2448–57.
125. Rizos H, Menzies AM, Pupo GM, et al. BRAF inhibitor resistance mechanisms in metastatic melanoma: spectrum and clinical impact. Clin Cancer Res 2014; 20(7):1965–77.
126. Wagle N, Emery C, Berger MF, et al. Dissecting therapeutic resistance to RAF inhibition in melanoma by tumor genomic profiling. J Clin Oncol 2011;29(22): 3085–96.
127. Shi H, Hong A, Kong X, et al. A novel AKT1 mutant amplifies an adaptive melanoma response to BRAF inhibition. Cancer Discov 2014;4(1):69–79.
128. Xing F, Persaud Y, Pratilas CA, et al. Concurrent loss of the PTEN and RB1 tumor suppressors attenuates RAF dependence in melanomas harboring (V600E) BRAF. Oncogene 2012;31(4):446–57.
129. Smalley KS, Lioni M, Dalla Palma M, et al. Increased cyclin D1 expression can mediate BRAF inhibitor resistance in BRAF V600E-mutated melanomas. Mol Cancer Ther 2008;7(9):2876–83.
130. Morris EJ, Jha S, Restaino CR, et al. Discovery of a novel ERK inhibitor with activity in models of acquired resistance to BRAF and MEK inhibitors. Cancer Discov 2013;3(7):742–50.
131. Sullivan RJ, Infante JR, Janku F, et al. First-in-Class ERK1/2 Inhibitor Ulixertinib (BVD-523) in Patients with MAPK mutant advanced solid tumors: results of a phase I dose-escalation and expansion study. Cancer Discov 2018;8(2):184–95.
132. Moschos SJ, Sullivan RJ, Hwu WJ, et al. Development of MK-8353, an orally administered ERK1/2 inhibitor, in patients with advanced solid tumors. JCI Insight 2018;3(4):e92352.
133. Schreuer M, Jansen Y, Planken S, et al. Combination of dabrafenib plus trametinib for BRAF and MEK inhibitor pretreated patients with advanced BRAF(V600)-mutant melanoma: an open-label, single arm, dual-centre, phase 2 clinical trial. Lancet Oncol 2017;18(4):464–72.
134. Das Thakur M, Salangsang F, Landman AS, et al. Modelling vemurafenib resistance in melanoma reveals a strategy to forestall drug resistance. Nature 2013; 494(7436):251–5.
135. Moriceau G, Hugo W, Hong A, et al. Tunable-combinatorial mechanisms of acquired resistance limit the efficacy of BRAF/MEK cotargeting but result in melanoma drug addiction. Cancer Cell 2015;27(2):240–56.
136. Algazi AP, Othus M, Daud AI, et al. Continuous versus intermittent BRAF and MEK inhibition in patients with BRAF-mutated melanoma: a randomized phase 2 trial. Nature Medicine 2020;26:1564–8.
137. Gay CM, Balaji K, Byers LA. Giving AXL the axe: targeting AXL in human malignancy. Br J Cancer 2017;116(4):415–23.

138. Zhu C, Wei Y, Wei X. AXL receptor tyrosine kinase as a promising anti-cancer approach: functions, molecular mechanisms and clinical applications. Mol Cancer 2019;18(1):153.
139. Boshuizen J, Koopman LA, Krijgsman O, et al. Cooperative targeting of melanoma heterogeneity with an AXL antibody-drug conjugate and BRAF/MEK inhibitors. Nat Med 2018;24(2):203–12.
140. Eroglu Z, Chen YA, Gibney GT, et al. Combined BRAF and HSP90 Inhibition in Patients with Unresectable BRAF (V600E)-Mutant Melanoma. Clin Cancer Res 2018;24(22):5516–24.

Cellular Therapy and Cytokine Treatments for Melanoma

Jessica S.W. Borgers, MD, John B.A.G. Haanen, MD, PhD*

KEYWORDS

- Melanoma • Adoptive cell therapy • TIL • TCR-T • CAR-T • Cytokines

KEY POINTS

- Adoptive cell transfer therapy using tumor-infiltrating lymphocytes has shown impressive results in patients with melanoma and is currently compared with standard-of-care ipilimumab in an ongoing phase III trial.
- The use of genetically modified T-cell receptor–engineered T cells and chimeric antigen receptor T cells in solid tumors is at its infancy and still faces many challenges.
- The use of recombinant cytokines has mostly been replaced with other treatments due to disappointing response rates and severe toxicities, although novel promising cytokine-based molecules are in clinical development.

INTRODUCTION

Despite breakthroughs in treatment of patients with advanced stage melanoma, mortality remains high. Cancer immunotherapy relies on the patient's immune system to recognize and eradicate the tumor. Cytokines are important immune mediators, as they serve as activation, inhibition, growth, and differentiation signals for a broad array of cells. In cancer treatment, recombinant cytokines have the potential to serve as immunomodulatory, antiproliferative and antiangiogenic agents. For many years, cytokines were the only US Food and Drug Administration (FDA)–approved treatments of patients with advanced stage melanoma. In the past decade, novel treatments including immune checkpoint inhibitors, small-molecule targeted therapies, and, more recently in clinical trial setting, adoptive cell transfer (ACT) treatments have mostly replaced the use of recombinant cytokines. ACT treatments using either tumor-infiltrating lymphocytes or engineered T cells have shown promising results in patients with melanoma with complete and durable responses.

Department of Medical Oncology, Netherlands Cancer Institute-Antoni van Leeuwenhoek, Plesmanlaan 121, Amsterdam 1066 CX, The Netherlands
* Corresponding author.
E-mail address: j.haanen@nki.nl

Hematol Oncol Clin N Am 35 (2021) 129–144
https://doi.org/10.1016/j.hoc.2020.08.014
0889-8588/21/© 2020 Elsevier Inc. All rights reserved.
hemonc.theclinics.com

In this review, the clinical experiences, results, toxicities, and future potential of adoptive cell therapies and recombinant cytokine treatments in melanoma are summarized.

Part I—Cellular Therapy

Tumor-infiltrating lymphocytes

Tumor-infiltrating lymphocytes (TIL) are autologous CD4+ and CD8+ T cells in the tumor microenvironment, which have the potential to recognize tumor-specific antigens.[1] However, because of chronic antigenic stimulation, they are converted to an "exhausted" state and become functionally impaired. In 1988, Rosenberg and colleagues[2] developed a method to reactivate these cells. By isolating autologous TIL from a resected metastasis, in vitro expansion in presence of interleukin (IL)-2 and reinfusion of the cells followed by IL-2 boluses, promising response rates were achieved.[2] TIL-production takes approximately one month and is successful in 75% to 97%.[3]

Based on previous studies that showed improved objective response rates (ORR) after lymphodepleting chemotherapy, patients are currently preconditioned before infusion with two days cyclophosphamide (60 mg/kg) followed by five days fludarabine (25 mg/m²).[2,4] This nonmyeloablative chemotherapy regimen is thought to enhance the antitumor efficacy of ACT by depletion of immunosuppressive cell populations and reduction of endogenous T cells, resulting in less competition for access to antigen-presenting cells and cytokines.[5] Common side effects of the chemotherapy are transient alopecia, nausea, pancytopenia, and febrile neutropenia.[1,4]

IL-2 plays an important role in the success of ACT. To support T-cell persistence and expansion in vivo after the TIL-infusion, patients subsequently receive IL-2 every 8 hours until tolerance, with a maximum of 15 doses.[6] The optimal dosing regimen is still unclear, although based on results from Goff and colleagues[7] the highest ORR seemed to be obtained after three to five high-dose (HD) IL-2 doses. IL-2 toxicities are dose related and include fever, chills, gastrointestinal tract symptoms, capillary leak syndrome, anemia, leukocytopenia, and thrombocytopenia.[8] Most of these are completely reversible on treatment discontinuation and can be managed using supportive measures.[8]

A recent meta-analysis by Dafni and colleagues[1] has found an ORR of 41% and a complete response rate (CRR) of 12% in a total of 410 patient treated with TIL. These percentages were higher in the HD IL-2 group than in the low-dose (LD) IL-2 group— 43% and 14%, compared with 35% and 7%, respectively.[1] This would favor the HD IL-2 regimen. The one-year overall survival (OS) rate in the HD IL-2 cohort was 56.5%.[1] Of the responders (complete response [CR], partial response [PR]) in this group, 55% progressed and 45% remained a responder after a median follow-up of 36 months.[1] When specifically looking at the patients with a CR, 14% of the HD IL-2 cohort, more than 90% remained in remission with a median follow-up of more than three years.[1]

Despite these promising results, TIL treatment has limitations: eligible patients need to have at least one resectable metastasis large enough to successfully grow TIL (1–3 cm in diameter), have a disease dynamic that allows delay of treatment of 5 to 7 weeks, and should be able to undergo the lymphodepleting chemotherapy and HD bolus IL-2 safely. Furthermore, the labor-intensive production requires highly specialized GMP facilities and qualified production staff.[3] Finally, the price per TIL treatment is relatively high, although a cost-effectiveness model favored TIL manufacture and treatment over ipilimumab.[9]

TIL has not yet been approved as standard-of-care treatment. A currently enrolling randomized phase III trial (NCT02278887) aims to show an improved survival rate after TIL-infusion compared to the standard-of-care ipilimumab in patients with advanced stage melanoma progressive on first-line anti-PD-1 treatment.

T-cell receptor–engineered T cells

Limitations of treatment with naturally occurring TIL, including the need for a surgically accessible metastasis and the laborious manufacturing process, have urged the development and utilization of genetically modified T cells: T-cell receptor–engineered T cells (TCR-T) and chimeric antigen receptor T cells (CAR-T) targeting specific tumor antigens.[10] TCR-T are manufactured from autologous PBMCs collected by apheresis, after which CD3+ cells are genetically modified and shortly expanded in vitro. After introduction of the TCR genes into the host genome, TCR-T are able to recognize antigenic peptides presented by major histocompatibility (MHC) molecules.[10] Potential targets for TCR-T are (1) shared melanoma-associated antigens, such as lineage antigens, cancer-testis antigens (CTA), overexpressed antigens, and (2) tumor-specific antigens including neoantigens.[11] Similar to TIL, patients are preconditioned by administration of lymphodepleting chemotherapy before infusion and, depending on the protocol, may receive IL-2 after infusion.[12,13]

In 2006, the first trial targeting the melanoma differentiation antigen MART-1 showed feasibility but only low clinical response rates (2/17).[12] More encouraging results were seen in subsequent trials with MART-1 and gp100 reactive TCR-T with objective tumor responses in 30% and 19% of patients, respectively.[13] Another trial combining MART-1 TCR-T with dendritic cell vaccination gave transient tumor regression in 9/13 patients.[14] Despite encouraging results, the downside of targeting antigens shared between melanoma cells and melanocytes is the risk of inducing "on-target, off-tumor toxicities." Destruction of melanocytes has led to severe skin toxicity, anterior uveitis, and ototoxicity in more than half of patients treated with these TCR-T.[13] These toxicities could be effectively treated with topical or systemic corticosteroids.[13,14]

Because of their very restricted expression on healthy tissues, CTA seem more attractive targets for TCR-T treatment.[15] However, these targets may be less safe than previously thought. In 2011, in two clinical trials targeting MAGE-A3 in multiple myeloma and melanoma, patients had unexpected fatal toxicities due to cross-reactivity with the heart protein titin and MAGE-A12 in the brain, respectively.[16,17] So far, no severe toxicities have been published after treatment with high-affinity NY-ESO-1-specific TCR gene–modified T cells, whereas encouraging response rates up to 55% and an estimated overall three- and five-year survival rate of 33% have been achieved in a phase II trial by Robbins and colleagues.[18]

Another strategy is by focusing on cancer neoantigens, genomic mutations, or aberrations in tumor cells that on gene expression may result in generation of novel antigenic peptides.[19] The advantage of exploiting these antigens is that these are completely foreign to the immune system and therefore are not subject to tolerance mechanisms.[19] Because of the tumor-specific nature of these mutations, the chance of cross-reactivity to normal tissue is minimal. The downside is that using neoantigen-specific TCRs requires a highly individualized manufacturing process, as every patient may require a unique set of neoantigen-specific TCRs. Another way of generating neoantigen-specific T cells that is currently tested is by inducing these cells from peripheral blood using neoantigen-specific stimulation, not requiring genetic modification (**Table 1**).

Table 1
Overview of ongoing adoptive cell therapy studies

NCT#	Intervention	Target	Condition	Phase	Status	Primary Outcome	Number to be Enrolled
TIL							
NCT04165967	TIL + LD IL-2 + nivolumab	-	Melanoma	I	Not yet recruiting	AEs, change in vital signs and full blood counts	9
NCT02278887	TIL vs ipilimumab	-	Melanoma	III	Recruiting	PFS	168
NCT03374839	TIL + HD IL-2 + nivolumab	-	Melanoma	I–II	Recruiting	AEs	11
NCT03475134	TIL + HD IL-2 + nivolumab	-	Melanoma	I	Recruiting	Feasibility, AEs	10
NCT03467516	TIL	-	Uveal melanoma	II	Recruiting	ORR	59
NCT02621021	TIL + HD IL-2 ± pembrolizumab	-	Melanoma	II	Recruiting	RR	170
NCT04217473	TILT-123 injection ± TIL	-	Melanoma	I	Recruiting	AEs, laboratory and vital sign abnormalities, ECG	15
NCT00604136	TIL + HD IL-2	-	Melanoma	II	Recruiting	RR	20
NCT03526185	TIL + LD IL-2 ± ipilimumab followed by nivolumab	-	Melanoma	Early I	Recruiting	AEs	30
NCT03166397	TIL + HD IL-2	-	Melanoma	II	Recruiting	ORR, AEs	30
NCT03638375	Nivolumab + TIL ± IFN-α	-	Melanoma	I–II	Recruiting	AEs	34
NCT00338377	TIL + HD IL-2 ± MART-1 DCs	MART-1	Melanoma, including leptomeningeal disease	II	Recruiting	irBOR, longitudinal immune response, ORR	189
NCT01955460	TGF-β-resistant (DNRII transduced) and NGFR-transduced TIL + HD IL-2	-	Melanoma	I	Recruiting	Feasibility and safety	15

NCT number	Treatment	Target	Cancer type	Phase	Status	Outcome measure	N
NCT03991741	TIL + HD IL-2	-	Melanoma, head and neck cancer	I	Recruiting	Dose-limiting toxicity	24
NCT04223648	Tremelimumab/durvalumab (1 cycle) + ipilimumab/nivolumab (3 cycles), if progression: PD-1 immunoselected TIL	-	Melanoma	Early I	Not yet recruiting	PD1+ cell pharmacodynamic response in blood to tremelimumab/durvalumab treatment	20
NCT03645928	TIL + IL-2 ± pembrolizumab	-	Melanoma, head and neck SCC, NSCLC	II	Recruiting	ORR, AEs	75
NCT02870244	1383I TCR transduced TIL + LD IL-2	Tyrosinase	Melanoma	I	Recruiting	AEs	18
NCT03997474	ATL001	Neoantigens	Melanoma	I-IIa	Recruiting	AEs	20
Blood-derived genetically enhanced T cells							
NCT04357509	Supercirculating TIL (ScTIL210)	Not specified	Melanoma	I	Not yet recruiting	ORR	32
Not yet known	NEO-PTC-01	Neoantigens	Melanoma	I	Not yet recruiting	Safety, MTD	26
TCR-T							
NCT03638206	NY-ESO TCR T cells	Multitarget, including NY-ESO-1	NY-ESO-1 expressing tumors, including melanoma	I-II	Recruiting	AEs	73
NCT03970382	NeoTCR-P1 T cells ± nivolumab	Neoantigens	Solid tumors, including melanoma	I	Recruiting	AEs, MTD, feasibility	148
NCT02650986	Autologous NY-ESO-1 TCR/dnTGFbetaRII transgenic T cells	NY-ESO-1	NY-ESO-1 expressing tumors, including melanoma	I-IIa	Recruiting	Safety and feasibility	27

(continued on next page)

Table 1
(continued)

NCT#	Intervention	Target	Condition	Phase	Status	Primary Outcome	Number to be Enrolled
NCT02869217	TBI-1301	NY-ESO-1	NY-ESO-1 expressing tumors, including melanoma	I	Recruiting	Safety, recommended phase II dose	22
NCT02111850	Anti-MAGE-A3-DP4 TCR cells	MAGE-A3	MAGE-A3 expressing tumors, including melanoma	I–II	Recruiting	Safety, RR, toxicity	107
NCT03133922	MAGE-A4[1032] T cells	MAGE-A4	MAGE-A4 expressing tumors, including melanoma	I	Recruiting	AEs, DLT, persistence of infused cells, RCL measurements in modified cells	42
NCT03649529	GPA-TriMAR-T	Gp100	Melanoma	Early I	Recruiting	Safety	6
CAR-T							
NCT03893019	MB-CART20.1	CD20	Melanoma	Early I	Recruiting	MTD, safety and toxicity	15
NCT03635632	C7R-GD2.CART cells	GD2	GD expressing tumors, including uveal melanoma	I	Recruiting	MTD	64

| NCT04119024 | Anti-hCD70 CART cells + HD IL-2 | CD70 | CD70 expressing tumors, including melanoma | I–II | Recruiting | AEs, RR | 124 |

Abbreviations: AEs, adverse events; CAR-T, chimeric antigen receptor T cells; DCs, dendritic cells; ECG, electrocardiogram; HD, high dose; IL-2, interleukin 2; IFN-α, interferon alpha; irBOR, immune-related best overall response; LD, low dose; MAGE, melanoma-associated antigen; MART-1, melanoma antigen recognized by T cells 1; MTD, maximum tolerated dose; NGFR, nerve growth factor receptor; NSCLC, non–small cell lung carcinoma; NY-ESO-1, New York esophageal squamous cell carcinoma 1; ORR, overall response rate; PD-1, programmed cell death protein 1; PFS, progression-free survival; RCL, replication-competent lentivirus; RR, response rate; SCC, squamous cell carcinoma; TCR-T, T cell receptor-engineered cells; TGF-β, transforming growth factor beta; TIL, tumor-infiltrating lymphocytes.

TCR gene therapy for the treatment of solid cancers is still at its infancy and faces many challenges. First, TCR-T recognize their target antigens as peptide-MHC complexes at the cell surface of tumor cells or antigen-presenting cells. In case of using a TCR directed at a shared tumor antigen, selection of patients requires human leukocyte antigen (HLA) typing and determining target protein expression by the tumor.[20] In addition, because of HLA and antigen expression dependency, tumors will attempt to escape T-cell–mediated responses by downregulation or loss of their HLA or antigen expression, resulting in a decrease of in vivo activity of the TCR-T.[21] Moreover, it is unlikely that targeting one single antigen will be sufficient to clear solid tumors.[20] Future studies targeting multiple antigens simultaneously may enhance the efficacy of TCR T cells in solid tumors, as has been shown in preclinical models.[22]

Chimeric antigen receptor T cells

To circumvent the need for HLA-dependent recognition of tumor cells, a limitation of TCR-T, CAR-T were developed. A CAR is a fully synthetic antigen receptor consisting of an antigen-binding site derived from an immunoglobulin, genetically linked to intracytoplasmic signaling molecules, including a CD3ζ-chain and either CD28 or CD137 (4-1BB) for costimulation.[23] CAR-T can be manufactured from both autologous and allogenic T cells, which are collected by apheresis, genetically modified to express the CAR and expanded over 7 to 10 days.[23] Similar to other ACTs in most solid cancer protocols, patients are preconditioned with a lymphodepleting regimen before infusion.

One of the advantages of CAR-T is their ability to recognize cell surface antigens in an MHC-independent manner.[23] As a consequence, they can be deployed to treat patients regardless of their HLA-type and can bypass tumor resistance mechanisms such as MHC downregulation and defective antigen processing.[21] As it is possible to knock-down the endogenous genes encoding TCRα/β chains and MHC I, patients can be treated with a universal, allogenic, "off-the-shelf" T-cell product,[24] which makes CAR-T an interesting alternative for patients who do not have an easily accessible tumor lesion or are in urgent need of treatment. An important limitation is that CAR-T can only recognize cell surface–expressed antigens, which are limited in number and often not tumor specific.

Their main successes so far have been in the field of hemato-oncology, whereas their efficacy against solid tumors remains unsatisfactory.[23,25] A phase I/II study testing vascular endothelial growth factor receptor 2 (VEGFR2) CAR-T (NCT01218867) in patients with metastatic cancer, including melanoma, was terminated due to lack of objective responses.[26] Currently, there are three phase I dose-escalation trials enrolling melanoma patients (see **Table 1**).

In order to enhance the efficacy of CAR-T for solid tumors, several challenges have to be overcome. The first is identifying the right target antigen. Most solid tumors lack antigens that are homogenously expressed and restricted to only tumor cells, thereby increasing the risk of "on-target, off-tumor" toxicity.[26] In addition, as for most T-cell immune interventions targeting a single antigen, development of antigen loss variants is an important obstacle.[27] Other challenges include inefficient trafficking and tumor infiltration and a hostile tumor microenvironment leading to suboptimal activation and survival of the engineered T cells.[23] Finally, compared with TIL, a high incidence of AEs has been observed. Two potentially lethal AEs are cytokine release syndrome (CRS) and immune effector cell–associated neurotoxicity syndrome (ICANS).[28] CRS is the result of in vivo activation and expansion of CAR T cells over the first 1 to 2 weeks after infusion and concurrent antigen recognition leading to massive cytokine release.[28] ICANS is thought to be associated with activation of central nervous endothelial cells and related increased permeability of the blood-brain barrier, leading to elevated cytokine levels in the central nervous system and cerebral infiltration by T cells.[29]

Part II—Cytokine Treatments

Interleukin-2

Interleukin-2 (IL-2) is a cytokine predominantly produced by activated CD4+ T cells and has paradoxic functions: it activates and promotes the proliferation of both anti-tumor effector CD8+ T cells, as well as suppressive CD4+ regulatory T cells (Tregs).[30] Despite these contradictory functions, the first trials using recombinant IL-2, aldesleukin, achieved an ORR of 16% and CRR of 6% in patients with advanced melanoma, leading to FDA approval in 1998.[31] Patients treated with IL-2 receive intravenously administrated boluses of 600,000 to 720,000 international units (IU)/kilogram (kg) every 8 hours for up to a maximum of 15 doses, with a second identical treatment cycle 6 to 9 days later.[31] This regimen can be repeated every 6 to 12 weeks in case of clinical response.[31] In a meta-analysis by Bright and colleagues[32] that included a total of 3312 patients, CRR was 4.0% (range 0%–23%), PRR 12.5%, and ORR was 19.7%.

The toxicities associated with recombinant IL-2 treatment limit its use in the clinic. Administration of IL-2 and subsequent activation of immune cells gives an abundant release of proinflammatory cytokines.[8] Furthermore, binding of IL-2 to the high-affinity IL-2Rα receptor expressed on endothelial cells results in capillary leak syndrome.[8] As a consequence, patients can experience symptoms including fever and chills, followed by hypotension, tachycardia, nausea, dyspnea, pulmonary edema, erythema, pruritus, and renal dysfunction.[8,31] The toxicities typically peak after 4 to 6 hours and often gradually subside before the following dose.[8] Most toxicities are preventable using premedication or can be effectively managed using supportive measures and are reversible after discontinuation of IL-2.[8] Because of these AEs, patients have to be hospitalized in experienced centers during treatment, making other treatment modalities such as targeted therapies or immune checkpoint inhibitors, which can be given in an ambulatory setting, more attractive as first- or second-line treatments.

In order to enhance the efficacy and reduce toxicities, alternative IL-2 structures have been and are being engineered. NKTR-214 (bempegaldesleukin) is a prodrug of recombinant IL-2 conjugated to six releasable polyethylene glycol (PEG) chains.[33] By PEGylating IL-2, the half-life is extended and the IL2Rα receptor binding ability is reduced, thereby decreasing its affinity for Tregs.[33] Several phase I/II and III trials are testing NKTR-214 both as monotherapy or in combination with immune checkpoint blockade (NCT03635983, NCT03138889). The preliminary results of the ongoing phase I/II PIVOT-02 study combining NKTR-214 with nivolumab (NCT02983045) are encouraging; of the 11 treatment-naive patients with advanced stage melanoma, a disease control rate of 91% and an ORR of 64% were observed, with very modest toxicities.[34] Similarly, BDG8, MDNA11, ALKS 4230 (NCT02799095), and THOR-707 (NCT04009681) also preferentially bind to the IL-2Rβγ dimer on effector cells and are undergoing preclinical and clinical testing. L19IL2 (Darleukin), a recombinant human L19 antibody specific to the alternatively spliced extradomain B domain of fibronectin (a marker of neoangiogenesis), fused to IL-2 enhances selective localization into the tumor.[35] The recently published results of a phase IIb trial (NCT01055522, recruitment 2010–2012) comparing dacarbazine monotherapy with the combination dacarbazine/L19IL2 in 69 patients with stage IV melanoma show a statistically significant benefit in ORR and median progression-free survival (PFS) for the combination treatment.[36] Currently, L19IL2 is being tested in combination with L19-TNF as neoadjuvant intralesional therapy in a phase III trial for patients with advanced stage melanoma (NCT03567889).

Interleukin-15

Both IL-2 and IL-15 promote CD8+ T and natural killer (NK) cell activation and proliferation, but, in contrast to IL-2, IL-15 has no effect on Tregs and does not cause capillary leak syndrome in preclinical models.[37] In the first-in-human phase I trial performed by Conlon and colleagues,[38] severe toxicities were seen after intravenous administration. Despite acceptable toxicities in a subsequent trial in which IL-15 was administered subcutaneously, stable disease was the best response observed.[39] In order to enhance the efficacy, IL-15/IL-15Rα complexes (ALT-803) were developed but without clinical benefit (NCT01727076).[40]

Despite disappointing clinical results, there is evidence that IL-7 and IL-15 may be superior to IL-2 when used in adoptive cell therapy.[41]

Interleukin-7

IL-7 plays an important role in the transition from effector to memory T cells and promotes recovery of lymphocytes after lymphodepletion.[42] Two phase I clinical trials have been performed in patients with metastatic melanoma. The first trial (NCT00091338), combining subcutaneously administered recombinant IL-7 with the melanoma peptides gp100 and MART-1, showed no objective responses.[43] Similar low response rates and acceptable toxicities were observed in the second trial (NCT00492440) in which patients were treated with escalating doses of subcutaneously administered recombinant IL-7.[44] There are currently no ongoing trials for patients with melanoma.

Interleukin-12

Based on functions such as activation of NK and cytotoxic T cells and inhibition of angiogenesis, this proinflammatory cytokine seemed an interesting anticancer agent.[45] After a promising phase I trial for melanoma and renal cell carcinoma (RCC) patients, unexpected severe toxicities were seen in the subsequent phase II trial, including two deaths.[46]

In order to increase cytokine concentrations in the tumor microenvironment and decrease systemic exposure, several strategies have been explored. The first strategy, intratumoral delivery of an IL-12 plasmid (tavokinogene telseplasmid [tavo]) by electroporation, was successful in a phase I trial (NCT00323206).[47] Further exploration in two phase II trials for patients with stage III/IV melanoma showed an ORR of 35.7% and a CRR of 17.9% as monotherapy with a median PFS of 3.7 months (NCT01502293).[48] In the second trial combining tavo with pembrolizumab in patients with immune desert tumors with low frequencies of checkpoint-positive TIL (NCT02493361), and of whom 42% has shown progression on anti-PD-1 treatment, encouraging results were found: 41%, 36%, 5.6 months, respectively.[49] A currently enrolling phase II trial, Keynote-695 (NCT03132675), aims to confirm these results. Second, the immunocytokine NHS-IL12, consisting of two IL-12 molecules fused to NHS76, an antibody with high affinity for both single- and double-stranded DNA which are exposed in necrotic tissue, has been developed to reduce systemic toxicity by selective delivery to the tumor.[50] This drug is being tested in two clinical trials for solid tumors: as monotherapy (NCT01417546) and in combination with avelumab (NCT02994953).

Interleukin-10

The administration of HD recombinant IL-10 or PEGylated IL-10 (pegilodecakin, AM0010) leads to activation, proliferation, and enhanced cytotoxicity of tumor-infiltrating CD8+ T cells, without inducing autoimmunity.[51] Based on results from the first-in-human phase I/Ib dose-escalation study for patients with advanced solid tumors, including four patients with melanoma, the recommended subcutaneous AM0010 dose for future studies was 20 µg/kg/d (NCT02009449).[52] The most common adverse events included anemia, thrombocytopenia, fatigue, fever, and injection site reactions; these were mostly transient. Of the patients with melanoma, one patient with ocular melanoma achieved a PR at least 72 weeks after treatment initiation, and one patient with cutaneous melanoma had an objective response in more than or equal to one lesion.[52] Subsequently, two phase II trials comparing the combination of pegilodecakin with pembrolizumab (NCT03382899) or nivolumab (NCT03382912) to monotherapy anti-PD-1 in patients with metastatic non–small cell lung cancer recently got closed early due to an unfavorable risk-benefit ratio. The results from a phase III trial for patients with metastatic pancreatic cancer are expected soon (NCT02923921).

Interleukin-21

IL-21 has been shown to boost antitumor immunity by enhancing CD8+ T and NK cell–mediated cytotoxicity and interferon (IFN)-γ production in preclinical studies, without stimulating the proliferation of T regs.[53] Clinical trials showed that IL-21 was well tolerated and induced cytokine production *in vivo*; however, there was limited efficacy as single agent or in combination with chemotherapy.[54,55] Adverse events included mild headache, fatigue, pyrexia, nausea, myalgia, rash, diarrhea, and injection site reactions; severe toxicities were mostly hematological and hepatic.[54,55] Two subsequent trials in metastatic RCC and metastatic colorectal cancer were terminated early due to severe toxicities and the finding that IL-21 plays a major role in promoting inflammation-induced colon cancer, respectively.[56,57] Consequently, direct administration of IL-21 was discontinued.

Interferon α

IFN-α became the first FDA-approved adjuvant treatment of high-risk stage IIB to stage III melanoma after successful completion of the Eastern Cooperative Oncology Group E1684 trial, in which IFN-α was compared with observation.[58] Using a treatment regimen of daily IV doses of 20 million units (MU)/m²/d for one month, followed by a maintenance period of subcutaneously administered doses of 10 MU/m² three times per week for 48 weeks, an increase in relapse-free survival (RFS; 20.6 vs 11.8 months) and OS (3.82 vs 2.78 years) was found in the IFN-α group.[58] Of the patients treated with this dosing regimen, the majority required dose modification or discontinuation due to severe adverse events.[58] Therefore, subsequent trials attempted to identify treatment regimens that would enhance the efficacy and lower the toxicities using both IFN-α and PEGylated IFN-α, which received FDA approval in 2011 after completion of the EORTC 18991 trial.[59] However, several systematic reviews and meta-analysis looking at the results of these trials only demonstrated an effect on RFS but no clear effects on OS.[60,61]

With the approval of targeted therapies and immune checkpoint inhibitors, which clearly show improved RFS in phase III studies and better tolerability, IFN-α as adjuvant treatment in stage III melanoma has become obsolete.

Granulocyte-macrophage colony-stimulating factor

The hematopoietic growth factor granulocyte-macrophage colony-stimulating factor (GM-CSF) seemed an interesting cytokine: it plays a role in the maturation and activation of dendritic cells, which in turn leads to the activation of T cells, and it stimulates the production of angiostatin, an angiogenesis suppressor, by tumor-infiltrating macrophages.[62] Numerous clinical trials have been performed testing recombinant GM-CSF as monotherapy or in combination with chemotherapy, cancer vaccines, or immune checkpoint inhibitors. Two studies performed by Spitler and colleagues[63,64] in which patients were treated with GM-CSF in 28-day cycles (125 μg/m^2 for 14 consecutive days) for 1 and 3 years provided the first evidence of the possible benefit of GM-CSF as adjuvant treatment, with a low rate of adverse events. Subsequent phase III trials by Lawson and colleagues[65,66] showed a trend toward improved RFS and OS in patients treated with GM-CSF compared with those treated with placebo, although not statistically significant. Ever since the completion of the phase III Oncovec (GM-CSF) Pivotal Trial in Melanoma in patients with stage IIIB to stage IVM1c comparing talimogene laherparepvec (T-VEC, modified herpes simplex virus encoding GM-CSF) with GM-CSF, which showed significant increases in durable response rates (16.3% vs 2.1%), ORR (26.4% vs 1.9%), and OS (23.3 vs 18.9 months) in the T-VEC treated arm, T-VEC became the preferred treatment option.[67]

SUMMARY

Immune checkpoint inhibitors and small-molecule targeted therapies (for BRAFV600E-mutated melanoma) have become the standard-of-care treatment options for advanced stage melanoma. However, as a large number of patients does not respond or becomes refractory to these treatments, the search for other agents continues. Historically, cytokine treatments were the first tested and, in case of IL-2 and TNF-α, FDA-approved treatments. Unfortunately, because of disappointing response rates and severe toxicities, their use has significantly decreased over recent years. More recently, ACT has proved to be a promising strategy with the ability to induce complete and durable remissions in patients with melanoma progressive on first-line treatment.

Ongoing and future trials testing modified cytokine constructs with enhanced pharmacodynamics and pharmacokinetics and adoptive cell therapies will help to optimize treatments for patients with advanced stage melanoma.

CLINICS CARE POINTS

- With an ORR of 41% and a CRR of 12%, TIL treatment is a promising new treatment modality for metastatic melanoma patients progressive upon the current standard of care treatments.
- Thus far, the disappointing clinical benefit and the high incidence of toxicities (including 'on-target, off-tumor' toxicities) have limited the use of TCR-T cells.
- The potential benefit of using CAR-T cells for the treatment of solid tumor is currently being explored. Special attention has to be paid to two potentially lethal adverse events: CRS and ICANS.
- Alternative structures of the cytokines IL-2 (NKTR-214, BDG8, MDNA11, ALKS 4230, THOR-707, L19IL2) and IL-12 (NHS-IL12) are currently being (pre)clinically tested in order to enhance the efficacy and reduce toxicities associated with cytokine treatments.

DISCLOSURE

J.B.A.G. Haanen has advisory roles for Achilles Therapeutics, AIMM, Amgen, Astra Zeneca, Bayer, BMS, Celsius Therapeutics, GSK, Immunocore, Ipsen, Merck Serono,

MSD, Neogene Therapeutics, Neon Therapeutics (BioNTech), Novartis, Pfizer, Roche/ Genentech, Sanofi, Seatlle Genetics, Third Rock Ventures, and Vaximm. J.B.A.G. Haanen received research grants from BMS, MSD, Neon Therapeutics, and Novartis.

REFERENCES

1. Dafni U, Michielin O, Lluesma SM, et al. Efficacy of adoptive therapy with tumor-infiltrating lymphocytes and recombinant interleukin-2 in advanced cutaneous melanoma: a systematic review and meta-analysis. Ann Oncol 2019;30(12):1902–13.

2. Rosenberg SA, Packard BS, Aebersold PM, et al. Use of tumor-infiltrating lymphocytes and interleukin-2 in the immunotherapy of patients with metastatic melanoma. A preliminary report. N Engl J Med 1988;319(25):1676–80.

3. Rohaan MW, van den Berg JH, Kvistborg P, et al. Adoptive transfer of tumor-infiltrating lymphocytes in melanoma: a viable treatment option. J Immunother Cancer 2018;6(1):102.

4. Dudley ME, Wunderlich JR, Yang JC, et al. Adoptive cell transfer therapy following non-myeloablative but lymphodepleting chemotherapy for the treatment of patients with refractory metastatic melanoma. J Clin Oncol 2005;23(10): 2346–57.

5. Muranski P, Boni A, Wrzesinski C, et al. Increased intensity lymphodepletion and adoptive immunotherapy–how far can we go? Nat Clin Pract Oncol 2006;3(12): 668–81.

6. Rosenberg SA, Yannelli JR, Yang JC, et al. Treatment of patients with metastatic melanoma with autologous tumor-infiltrating lymphocytes and interleukin 2. J Natl Cancer Inst 1994;86(15):1159–66.

7. Goff SL, Dudley ME, Citrin DE, et al. Randomized, prospective evaluation comparing intensity of lymphodepletion before adoptive transfer of tumor-infiltrating lymphocytes for patients with metastatic melanoma. J Clin Oncol 2016;34(20):2389–97.

8. Marabondo S, Kaufman HL. High-dose interleukin-2 (IL-2) for the treatment of melanoma: safety considerations and future directions. Expert Opin Drug Saf 2017;16(12):1347–57.

9. Retel VP, Steuten LM, Mewes JC, et al. Early cost-effectiveness modeling for tumor infiltrating lymphocytes (TIL) -treatment versus ipilimumab in metastatic melanoma patients. Value Health 2014;17(7):A640.

10. Houot R, Schultz LM, Marabelle A, et al. T-cell-based immunotherapy: adoptive cell transfer and checkpoint inhibition. Cancer Immunol Res 2015;3(10):1115–22.

11. Pitcovski J, Shahar E, Aizenshtein E, et al. Melanoma antigens and related immunological markers. Crit Rev Oncol Hematol 2017;115:36–49.

12. Morgan RA, Dudley ME, Wunderlich JR, et al. Cancer regression in patients after transfer of genetically engineered lymphocytes. Science 2006;314(5796):126–9.

13. Johnson LA, Morgan RA, Dudley ME, et al. Gene therapy with human and mouse T-cell receptors mediates cancer regression and targets normal tissues expressing cognate antigen. Blood 2009;114(3):535–46.

14. Chodon T, Comin-Anduix B, Chmielowski B, et al. Adoptive transfer of MART-1 T-cell receptor transgenic lymphocytes and dendritic cell vaccination in patients with metastatic melanoma. Clin Cancer Res 2014;20(9):2457–65.

15. Simpson AJ, Caballero OL, Jungbluth A, et al. Cancer/testis antigens, gametogenesis and cancer. Nat Rev Cancer 2005;5(8):615–25.

16. Linette GP, Stadtmauer EA, Maus MV, et al. Cardiovascular toxicity and titin cross-reactivity of affinity-enhanced T cells in myeloma and melanoma. Blood 2013; 122(6):863–71.

17. Morgan RA, Chinnasamy N, Abate-Daga D, et al. Cancer regression and neurological toxicity following anti-MAGE-A3 TCR gene therapy. J Immunother 2013; 36(2):133–51.

18. Robbins PF, Kassim SH, Tran TL, et al. A pilot trial using lymphocytes genetically engineered with an NY-ESO-1-reactive T-cell receptor: long-term follow-up and correlates with response. Clin Cancer Res 2015;21(5):1019–27.

19. Schumacher TN, Schreiber RD. Neoantigens in cancer immunotherapy. Science 2015;348(6230):69–74.

20. Garber K. Driving T-cell immunotherapy to solid tumors. Nat Biotechnol 2018; 36(3):215–9.

21. Garrido F, Ruiz-Cabello F, Aptsiauri N. Rejection versus escape: the tumor MHC dilemma. Cancer Immunol Immunother 2017;66(2):259–71.

22. Kaluza KM, Kottke T, Diaz RM, et al. Adoptive transfer of cytotoxic T lymphocytes targeting two different antigens limits antigen loss and tumor escape. Hum Gene Ther 2012;23(10):1054–64.

23. Muhammad N, Mao Q, Xia H. CAR T-cells for cancer therapy. Biotechnol Genet Eng Rev 2017;33(2):190–226.

24. Poirot L, Philip B, Schiffer-Mannioui C, et al. Multiplex genome-edited T-cell manufacturing platform for "off-the-shelf" adoptive t-cell immunotherapies. Cancer Res 2015;75(18):3853–64.

25. D'Aloia MM, Zizzari IG, Sacchetti B, et al. CAR-T cells: the long and winding road to solid tumors. Cell Death Dis 2018;9(3):282.

26. Li H, Zhao Y. Increasing the safety and efficacy of chimeric antigen receptor T cell therapy. Protein & cell 2017;8(8):573–89.

27. Olson BM, McNeel DG. Antigen loss and tumor-mediated immunosuppression facilitate tumor recurrence. Expert Rev Vaccines 2012;11(11):1315–7.

28. Brudno JN, Kochenderfer JN. Toxicities of chimeric antigen receptor T cells: recognition and management. Blood 2016;127(26):3321–30.

29. Gust J, Hay KA, Hanafi LA, et al. Endothelial activation and blood-brain barrier disruption in neurotoxicity after adoptive immunotherapy with CD19 CAR-T Cells. Cancer Discov 2017;7(12):1404–19.

30. Boyman O, Sprent J. The role of interleukin-2 during homeostasis and activation of the immune system. Nat Rev Immunol 2012;12(3):180–90.

31. Atkins MB, Lotze MT, Dutcher JP, et al. High-dose recombinant interleukin 2 therapy for patients with metastatic melanoma: analysis of 270 patients treated between 1985 and 1993. J Clin Oncol 1999;17(7):2105–16.

32. Bright R, Coventry BJ, Eardley-Harris N, et al. Clinical response rates from interleukin-2 therapy for metastatic melanoma over 30 years' experience: a meta-analysis of 3312 patients. J Immunother 2017;40(1):21–30.

33. Doberstein SK. Bempegaldesleukin (NKTR-214): a CD-122-biased IL-2 receptor agonist for cancer immunotherapy. Expert Opin Biol Ther 2019;19(12):1223–8.

34. Ascierto PA, Flaherty K, Goff S. Emerging strategies in systemic therapy for the treatment of melanoma. Am Soc Clin Oncol Educ Book 2018;38:751–8.

35. Carnemolla B, Borsi L, Balza E, et al. Enhancement of the antitumor properties of interleukin-2 by its targeted delivery to the tumor blood vessel extracellular matrix. Blood 2002;99(5):1659–65.

36. Weide B, Eigentler T, Catania C, et al. A phase II study of the L19IL2 immunocytokine in combination with dacarbazine in advanced metastatic melanoma patients. Cancer Immunol Immunother 2019;68(9):1547–59.
37. Waldmann TA, Lugli E, Roederer M, et al. Safety (toxicity), pharmacokinetics, immunogenicity, and impact on elements of the normal immune system of recombinant human IL-15 in rhesus macaques. Blood 2011;117(18):4787–95.
38. Conlon KC, Lugli E, Welles HC, et al. Redistribution, hyperproliferation, activation of natural killer cells and CD8 T cells, and cytokine production during first-in-human clinical trial of recombinant human interleukin-15 in patients with cancer. J Clin Oncol 2015;33(1):74–82.
39. Miller JS, Morishima C, McNeel DG, et al. A first-in-human phase i study of subcutaneous outpatient recombinant human IL15 (rhIL15) in Adults with Advanced Solid Tumors. Clin Cancer Res 2018;24(7):1525–35.
40. Margolin K, Morishima C, Velcheti V, et al. Phase I Trial of ALT-803, A novel recombinant il15 complex, in patients with advanced solid tumors. Clin Cancer Res 2018;24(22):5552–61.
41. Kaneko S, Mastaglio S, Bondanza A, et al. IL-7 and IL-15 allow the generation of suicide gene-modified alloreactive self-renewing central memory human T lymphocytes. Blood 2009;113(5):1006–15.
42. Lin J, Zhu Z, Xiao H, et al. The role of IL-7 in Immunity and Cancer. Anticancer Res 2017;37(3):963–7.
43. Rosenberg SA, Sportes C, Ahmadzadeh M, et al. IL-7 administration to humans leads to expansion of CD8+ and CD4+ cells but a relative decrease of CD4+ T-regulatory cells. J Immunother 2006;29(3):313–9.
44. Sportes C, Babb RR, Krumlauf MC, et al. Phase I study of recombinant human interleukin-7 administration in subjects with refractory malignancy. Clin Cancer Res 2010;16(2):727–35.
45. Perussia B, Chan SH, D'Andrea A, et al. Natural killer (NK) cell stimulatory factor or IL-12 has differential effects on the proliferation of TCR-alpha beta+, TCR-gamma delta+ T lymphocytes, and NK cells. J Immunol 1992;149(11):3495–502.
46. Leonard JP, Sherman ML, Fisher GL, et al. Effects of single-dose interleukin-12 exposure on interleukin-12-associated toxicity and interferon-gamma production. Blood 1997;90(7):2541–8.
47. Daud AI, DeConti RC, Andrews S, et al. Phase I trial of interleukin-12 plasmid electroporation in patients with metastatic melanoma. J Clin Oncol 2008;26(36): 5896–903.
48. Algazi A, Bhatia S, Agarwala S, et al. Intratumoral delivery of tavokinogene telseplasmid yields systemic immune responses in metastatic melanoma patients. Ann Oncol 2020;31(4):532–40.
49. Algazi AP, Twitty CG, Tsai KK, et al. Phase II Trial of IL-12 Plasmid Transfection and PD-1 Blockade in Immunologically Quiescent Melanoma. Clin Cancer Res 2020;26(12):2827–37.
50. Fallon J, Tighe R, Kradjian G, et al. The immunocytokine NHS-IL12 as a potential cancer therapeutic. Oncotarget 2014;5(7):1869–84.
51. Naing A, Infante JR, Papadopoulos KP, et al. PEGylated IL-10 (Pegilodecakin) induces systemic immune activation, CD8(+) T Cell invigoration and polyclonal T cell expansion in cancer patients. Cancer Cell 2018;34(5):775–91.e3.
52. Naing A, Papadopoulos KP, Autio KA, et al. Safety, antitumor activity, and immune activation of pegylated recombinant human interleukin-10 (AM0010) in patients with advanced solid tumors. J Clin Oncol 2016;34(29):3562–9.

53. Skak K, Kragh M, Hausman D, et al. Interleukin 21: combination strategies for cancer therapy. Nat Rev Drug Discov 2008;7(3):231–40.
54. Davis ID, Brady B, Kefford RF, et al. Clinical and biological efficacy of recombinant human interleukin-21 in patients with stage IV malignant melanoma without prior treatment: a phase IIa trial. Clin Cancer Res 2009;15(6):2123–9.
55. Petrella TM, Tozer R, Belanger K, et al. Interleukin-21 has activity in patients with metastatic melanoma: a phase II study. J Clin Oncol 2012;30(27):3396–401.
56. Grünwald V, Desar IM, Haanen J, et al. A phase I study of recombinant human interleukin-21 (rIL-21) in combination with sunitinib in patients with metastatic renal cell carcinoma (RCC). Acta Oncol 2011;50(1):121–6.
57. Steele N, Anthony A, Saunders M, et al. A phase 1 trial of recombinant human IL-21 in combination with cetuximab in patients with metastatic colorectal cancer. Br J Cancer 2012;106(5):793–8.
58. Kirkwood JM, Strawderman MH, Ernstoff MS, et al. Interferon alfa-2b adjuvant therapy of high-risk resected cutaneous melanoma: the Eastern Cooperative Oncology Group Trial EST 1684. J Clin Oncol 1996;14(1):7–17.
59. Eggermont AM, Suciu S, Testori A, et al. Long-term results of the randomized phase III trial EORTC 18991 of adjuvant therapy with pegylated interferon alfa-2b versus observation in resected stage III melanoma. J Clin Oncol 2012; 30(31):3810–8.
60. Wheatley K, Ives N, Eggermont A, et al. Interferon-α as adjuvant therapy for melanoma: An individual patient data meta-analysis of randomised trials. J Clin Oncol 2007;25(18_suppl):8526.
61. Mocellin S, Lens MB, Pasquali S, et al. Interferon alpha for the adjuvant treatment of cutaneous melanoma. Cochrane Database Syst Rev 2013;(6):CD008955.
62. Shi Y, Liu CH, Roberts AI, et al. Granulocyte-macrophage colony-stimulating factor (GM-CSF) and T-cell responses: what we do and don't know. Cell Res 2006; 16(2):126–33.
63. Spitler LE, Grossbard ML, Ernstoff MS, et al. Adjuvant therapy of stage III and IV malignant melanoma using granulocyte-macrophage colony-stimulating factor. J Clin Oncol 2000;18(8):1614–21.
64. Spitler LE, Weber RW, Allen RE, et al. Recombinant human granulocyte-macrophage colony-stimulating factor (GM-CSF, sargramostim) administered for 3 years as adjuvant therapy of stages II(T4), III, and IV melanoma. J Immunother 2009;32(6):632–7.
65. Lawson DH, Lee SJ, Tarhini AA, et al. E4697: Phase III cooperative group study of yeast-derived granulocyte macrophage colony-stimulating factor (GM-CSF) versus placebo as adjuvant treatment of patients with completely resected stage III-IV melanoma. J Clin Oncol 2010;28(15_suppl):8504.
66. Lawson DH, Lee S, Zhao F, et al. Randomized, placebo-controlled, phase III trial of yeast-derived granulocyte-macrophage colony-stimulating factor (GM-CSF) Versus Peptide Vaccination Versus GM-CSF Plus Peptide Vaccination Versus Placebo in Patients With No Evidence of Disease After Complete Surgical Resection of Locally Advanced and/or Stage IV Melanoma: A Trial of the Eastern Cooperative Oncology Group-American College of Radiology Imaging Network Cancer Research Group (E4697). J Clin Oncol 2015;33(34):4066–76.
67. Andtbacka RH, Kaufman HL, Collichio F, et al. Talimogene laherparepvec improves durable response rate in patients with advanced melanoma. J Clin Oncol 2015;33(25):2780–8.

Combinatorial Approaches to the Treatment of Advanced Melanoma

Rodrigo Ramella Munhoz, MD[a],*, Michael Andrew Postow, MD[b]

KEYWORDS

- Melanoma • BRAF • Immunotherapy • MAPK

KEY POINTS

- Monoclonal antibodies targeting immune-checkpoints (ICP) and BRAF/MEK inhibitors result in robust antitumor activity in melanoma - nevertheless, a significant proportion of patients exhibit primary or secondary resistance.
- Combinatorial approaches may result in increased activity and more durable responses in advanced melanoma, and this has been demonstrated with regimens combining different ICP blockers and BRAF/MEK inhibitors.
- The growing number of agents under clinical development may expand the clinical use of combinatorial approaches in melanoma.

INTRODUCTION

Melanoma corresponds to most deaths attributable to skin malignancies worldwide. Updated estimates suggest approximately 60,000 new cases in men and 40,000 new cases in women will be diagnosed in 2020, a surge in incidence over the past 20 years.[1,2]

Although still a challenging disease, treatment of advanced melanoma has made remarkable progress in the past decade with significant improvement in its historically dismal long-term survival outcomes. The characterization of molecules that contribute to immune evasion by downregulating T-cell–mediated antitumor responses led to the development of immune-checkpoint blockade (ICB), exemplified by strategies that inhibit cytotoxic T-lymphocyte–associated antigen 4 (CTLA4) and programmed cell death protein 1 (PD1) and its ligand (PD-L1).[3] Monoclonal antibodies against CTLA-4 and PD-1, capable of restoring antitumor immunity and reversing T-cell exhaustion, demonstrated robust antitumor activity and sustained responses in patients with

Funding: No funding received.
[a] Oncology Center, Hospital Sírio Libanês, Rua Dona Adma Jafet, 91, São Paulo 01308-050, Brazil; [b] Melanoma Service, Memorial Sloan Kettering Cancer Center, Weill Cornell Medical College, 1275 York Avenue, New York, NY 10065, USA
* Corresponding author.
E-mail address: rodrigo.rmunhoz@hsl.org.br

Hematol Oncol Clin N Am 35 (2021) 145–158
https://doi.org/10.1016/j.hoc.2020.08.015
0889-8588/21/© 2020 Elsevier Inc. All rights reserved.

hemonc.theclinics.com

advanced melanoma.[4] In addition to ICB, a distinct form of immunotherapy, talimogene laherparepvec (T-VEC), an oncolytic attenuated herpes simplex virus-1, induces antitumor responses by selectively replicating and lysing tumor cells while overexpressing granulocyte macrophage colony-stimulating factor (GM-CSF) to boost an immune response.[5] Concurrent with these advances in immunotherapy, the prominent role-activating mutations involving the V-Raf Murine Sarcoma Viral Oncogene Homolog B (BRAF) gene play in approximately 50% of patients paved the way for the development of targeted therapies that block components of the mitogen-activated protein kinase pathway (MAPK) signaling pathway. As a result, the ICB blockers ipilimumab, nivolumab, and pembrolizumab, the oncolytic virus T-VEC, and molecules targeting the MAPK pathway have been approved by the Food and Drug Administration (FDA) and incorporated into clinical practice.[4]

The efficacy of these therapies, however, can be hampered by primary and secondary resistance mechanisms, resulting in poor or transient responses in a significant proportion of patients with advanced melanoma. In this scenario of unmet clinical need, combined approaches have emerged as an alternative to enhance the benefit of systemic treatments. Regimens consisting of combined ICB blockers and separately, BRAF and mitogen-activated protein kinase kinase (MEK) inhibitors are now part of the available armamentarium. However, improvements in antitumor activity through combinations may come at a cost of incremental toxicities or financial burden, and weighing the magnitude of benefit in the face of multiple treatment options is crucial for balanced treatment decisions.

In this article, we first review highlights of data for single agents to provide a context to understand the efficacy of combinatorial approaches in melanoma, including the currently approved combinations of immune-checkpoint blockers and combined BRAF and MEK inhibitors (**Table 1**). We then discuss emerging strategies using multimodality regimens for the treatment of advanced melanoma. Given the high number of combinations under investigation, we focus exclusively on combinations that are approved by regulatory agencies in clinical use or combinations in large phase 3 randomized studies for the treatment of patients with unresectable stage III or IV melanoma.

FIRST-LINE MONOTHERAPY REGIMENS IN MELANOMA AS A BACKGROUND TO UNDERSTANDING EFFICACY OF COMBINATIONS

The incorporation of monoclonal antibodies capable of inhibiting negative coreceptors in the immune synapse and reversing immune-tolerance and T-cell exhaustion mechanisms, initially through the anti–CTLA-4 agent ipilimumab, and subsequently though PD-1 blockers, represented a major breakthrough in the management of advanced melanoma. Following initial survival gains resulting from ipilimumab, a series of studies demonstrated even more robust antitumor activity with both nivolumab and pembrolizumab as single agents. Despite the need for more efficacious approaches, single-agent ICB with either nivolumab or pembrolizumab remains standard first-line treatment for patients with advanced melanoma.

In recent updates with long-term follow-up of phase I clinical trials, both nivolumab and pembrolizumab demonstrated objective response rates (ORR) of approximately 30%, with almost 34% of the patients alive at 5 years.[6,7] When used in immunotherapy-naïve patients, which corresponds to a current indication for anti–PD-1 agents, both pembrolizumab and nivolumab showed superiority in terms of ORR, progression-free survival (PFS), overall survival (OS), and tolerability when compared to ipilimumab. The activity of first-line, single-agent nivolumab was demonstrated in 2

Table 1
Summary of selected, pivotal randomized clinical trials addressing combinatorial approaches for the treatment of patients with advanced melanoma

Study	Author/Year	Regimen[a]	ORR[a]	PFS/OS[a]	AEs[a] (Grade 3 or Higher)
Combined immune-checkpoint blockade					
CM-069	Postow et al.[18] 2015	IPI 3 mg/kg + NIVO 1 mg/kg -> NIVO 3 mg/kg	61%[c]	NR	54%
CM-067	Larkin et al.[9] 2019	IPI 3 mg/kg + NIVO 1 mg/kg -> NIVO 3 mg/kg	58%	Median PFS: 11.5 m/5y OS: 52%	59%
CM-511	Lebbé et al,[22] 2019	IPI 1 mg/kg + NIVO 3 mg/kg	45.6%	Median PFS: 9.9 m	34%
Combined BRAF and MEK inhibitors[b]					
COMBI-v[b] COMBI-d[b]	Robert et al,[25] 2019	Dabrafenib 150 mg bid + Trametinib 2 mg qd	68%	Median PFS: 11.1 m/Median OS: 25.9 m	59%
coBRIM[b]	Dréno et al.[26] 2018	Vemurafenib 960 mg bid + Cobimetinib 60 mg qd	70%	Median OS: 22.5 m	77%
COLUMBUS[b]	Dummer et al.[27] 2018	Encorafenib 450 mg QD + Binimetinib 45 mg BID	63% (central review)	Median PFS: 14.9 m/Median OS: 33.6 m	64%
Combined IT and TT					
KEYNOTE-022[b]	Ascierto et al.[39] 2019	Pembrolizumab 2 mg/kg q3w + Dabrafenib 150 mg BID + Trametinib 2 mg QD	-	Median PFS: 16m	58.3%
TRILOGY[b]	McArthur et al. 2020	Vemurafenib 720 mg BID + Cobimetinib 60 mg QD + Atezolizumab 840 mg q14 d	66.3%	Median PFS: 16.1 m/median OS 28.8 m	-

Abbreviations: AEs, incidence of grade 3 or higher adverse events; BID, twice daily; IPI, ipilimumab; IT, immunotherapy; NIVO, nivolumab; NR, not reached; ORR, objective response rate; OS, overall survival; PFS, progression-free survival; QD, once daily; TT, targeted therapy.
[a] In treatment arms comprising combinations.
[b] Trials limited to patients with tumors harboring a BRAF B600 E or V600 K mutation.
[c] Among patients with BRAF wild-type tumors.

randomized trials, CheckMate-066 (limited to patients with BRAF wild-type tumors, in comparison to chemotherapy) and CheckMate-067 (in comparison to ipilimumab).[8,9] In the first study, nivolumab resulted in an ORR of 42.8% and a median OS of 37.5 months, with 15% of the patients developing grade 3 or 4 adverse events (AEs). In CheckMate-067, median OS was 36.9 months, with a 5-year OS rate of 44%. In the phase III KEYNOTE-006 trial, patients were randomized to 2 dosing regimens of pembrolizumab administered every 3 weeks, or ipilimumab 3 mg/kg every 3 weeks for 4 doses. After a median follow-up of 57.7 months, pembrolizumab resulted in a significant improvement in OS (median OS: 32.7 m vs 15.9 m; hazard ratio 0.73; $P = .00049$) and a favorable toxicity profile, with an incidence of treatment-related grade 3 to 4 AEs of 17%. In the combined treatment-naïve cohorts treated with pembrolizumab, median OS was 38.7 months, with 43.2% of the patients alive at 5 years.[10]

In addition to ICB, MAPK pathway blockade has proven to be an important approach for the treatment of advanced melanoma in patients with BRAF mutations. The BRAF inhibitors vemurafenib and dabrafenib demonstrated striking activity in randomized trials, with ORR approaching 50%. Nevertheless, the onset of secondary resistance resulted in short-lived disease control, resulting in median PFS intervals approaching 7 months and a median OS of approximately 14 months. Long-term benefit was limited to a small proportion of patients.[11,12] With the development of superior approaches that combined BRAF and MEK inhibitors, the use of single-agent BRAF inhibitors is no longer acceptable, unless patients have specific contraindications to MEK inhibitors, such as a low cardiac ejection fraction or poor eyesight.

COMBINATORIAL APPROACHES IN ADVANCED MELANOMA
Combinations of Immune-Checkpoint Blockers

The combination of ipilimumab with nivolumab was initially interrogated in a phase 1 trial that included 86 patients with advanced melanoma and was based on the rationale that CTLA-4 and PD-1 modulate distinct, nonredundant immunologic mechanisms of escape from immune surveillance. Supporting preclinical evidence additionally suggested enhanced, and potentially synergistic activity with dual ICB blockade.[13,14] The phase 1 study consisted of 53 patients receiving escalating doses of concurrent ipilimumab combined with nivolumab administered every 3 weeks for 4 doses, followed by single-agent nivolumab every 3 weeks for 4 doses, and subsequently the combined treatment every 12 weeks for up to 8 doses. The ORR in these initial concurrent cohorts according to modified World Health Organization criteria was 40%; treatment-related grade 3 or 4 AEs were noted in 53%. In dose escalation, both nivolumab 1 mg/kg + ipilimumab 3 mg/kg and nivolumab 3 mg/kg + ipilimumab 1 mg/kg had similar rates of efficacy and toxicity. It was therefore difficult to determine the best dose to advance for clinical development. Given dose dependent efficacy for ipilimumab as monotherapy and no clear dose dependency of single-agent anti-PD1 agents along with knowledge that only ipilimumab 3 mg/kg had an established OS benefit, the nivolumab 1 mg/kg + ipilimumab 3 mg/kg regimen was chosen for phase 2 and 3 study.[15–17]

Two subsequent trials led to the approval by the FDA in 2015 of the combination of ipilimumab and nivolumab for patients with advanced melanoma. CheckMate-069 was a double-blind, randomized phase II study that included 142 treatment-naïve patients who received ipilimumab 3 mg/kg combined nivolumab 1 mg/kg or placebo every 3 weeks for 4 doses, followed by nivolumab 3 mg/kg or placebo every 2 weeks until disease progression or unacceptable toxicity.[18] The primary endpoint was the rate of objective responses among individuals with BRAF wild-type tumors, which corresponded to approximately 75% of the study population. In this subgroup, the ORR was 61% for the combination (similar to those with BRAF-mutant tumors) versus 11% for those receiving ipilimumab alone (P<.001). Treatment-related AEs of grades 3 or 4 occurred in 54% of the patients treated with the combination. In a subsequent publication of longer-term results, with a median follow-up 24.5 months, the 2-year OS rate in the combination arm was 63.8%.[19]

The pivotal CheckMate-067 study that confirmed the efficacy of ipilimumab + nivolumab was a 3-arm, double-blind, randomized trial in which 945 patients with unresectable stage III or stage IV melanoma were randomized in a 1:1:1 ratio to receive nivolumab 1 mg/kg plus ipilimumab 3 mg/kg every 3 weeks for 4 doses followed by nivolumab every 2 weeks, nivolumab 3 mg/kg plus placebo every 2 weeks, or ipilimumab 3 mg/kg plus placebo.[20] The study was designed to compare the nivolumab-containing arms with single-agent ipilimumab, with PFS and OS as co-primary endpoints; the direct comparison of the combination versus single-agent nivolumab was exploratory. Patients were stratified according to tumor PD-L1 expression, BRAF V600 mutation status and American Joint Committee on Cancer stage. Following initial demonstration of improvement in PFS for the nivolumab-containing arms versus ipilimumab, the 5-year outcomes in this trial have been recently updated.[9] The median OS has not been reached for the ipilimumab and nivolumab group (more than 60 months), and was 36.9 months and 19.9 months for single-agent nivolumab or ipilimumab, respectively, with an apparent plateau on survival curves at 3 years after treatment initiation. The 5-year OS rate was 52% among patients treated with combination, 44% in the nivolumab group and 26% in the ipilimumab group, with 5-year PFS rates of 36%, 29%, and 8%, respectively. Fifty-eight percent of those receiving ipilimumab plus nivolumab achieved an objective response versus 45% in the nivolumab group and 19% in the ipilimumab group. Grade 3 and 4 AEs for the combination, nivolumab alone, and ipilimumab alone were 59%, 23%, and 28%, respectively, and 42% of the patients discontinued treatment due to toxicities in the combination arm, versus 13% with single-agent nivolumab.[9]

The high incidence of immune-related AEs has been a major concern with the use of combined ICB blockade, and efforts have focused on alternative strategies to mitigate these toxicities. In the phase 1b KEYNOTE-029 trial, 153 patients were treated with a regimen consisting of "low-dose" ipilimumab (1 mg/kg) combined with standard dose of pembrolizumab 2 mg/kg given every 3 weeks for 4 doses, followed by single-agent pembrolizumab for up to 2 years. The ORR in this study was 57%, with 89% of the patients alive at 12 months. Grade 3 to 4 AEs occurred in 45% of the cases, with toxicities leading to treatment discontinuation in only 14% of the patients.[21] Although nonrandomized, these data were the first to suggest lower dose ipilimumab + anti-PD1 may have similar efficacy with lower toxicity as the higher ipilimumab dose regimens in combination with anti-P1.

To more formally explore this essential dosing question, the randomized CheckMate-511 study tested whether ipilimumab 1 mg/kg in combination with nivolumab 3 mg/kg reduced incidence of severe AEs in comparison to the standard dosing of the combination regimen, ipilimumab 3 mg/kg + nivolumab 1 mg/kg.[22] The primary endpoint was the rate of treatment-related grade 3 to 5 AEs; ORR, PFS, OS and health-related quality of life were secondary outcomes. The alternative dosing regimen of ipilimumab 1 mg/kg and nivolumab 3 mg/kg resulted in a reduced incidence of grade 3 to 5 AEs (34% vs 48%; P = .006), largely influenced by lower rates of hepatic, gastrointestinal, and endocrine toxicities. Efficacy, although a descriptive comparison only, because the study was not designed as a noninferiority trial, did not appear different between the ipilimumab 1 mg/kg and 3 mg/kg arms, respectively (ORR 45.6% vs 50.6%, median PFS 9.9 m vs 8.9 m, median OS not reached in both arms).[22] Longer follow-up of this study will be needed to truly understand whether lower doses of ipilimumab are as apparently effective as the standard dose of this combination.

Combinations of V-Raf Murine Sarcoma Viral Oncogene Homolog B and Mitogen-Activated Protein Kinase Kinase Inhibitors in V-Raf Murine Sarcoma Viral Oncogene Homolog B–Mutant Melanoma

As previously highlighted, despite initial response, secondary resistance, largely attributable to the reactivation of the MAPK pathway in 70% of cases, often limits the benefit of single-agent BRAF inhibitors.[23] Hence, a multitargeted approach, with combined blockade of downstream signaling components through the addition of a MEK inhibitor emerged as an option with the capability to delay treatment resistance and enhance the antitumor effect of targeted therapy. In addition, this strategy was developed to reduce toxicities related to the use of single-agent BRAF inhibitors that resulted from paradoxic activation of the MAPK pathway, particularly hyperkeratosis and second-primary cutaneous malignancies (keratoacanthomas and squamous-cell carcinomas). Following early evidence that simultaneous, rather than sequential administration of BRAF and MEK inhibitors could optimize the antitumor effect, 4 randomized, phase 3 studies confirmed the superiority in terms of ORR, PFS, and OS of BRAF inhibitors (vemurafenib, dabrafenib, or encorafenib) administered concurrently with MEK inhibitors (cobimetinib, trametinib, or binimetinib) in comparison with single-agent BRAF inhibitors, resulting in the approval by the FDA of 3 doublets.

The combination dabrafenib (150 mg twice daily continuously) plus trametinib (2 mg once daily continuously) was compared with single-agent dabrafenib or vemurafenib in the COMBI-d and COMBI-v trials, respectively, with ORRs approaching 70% and a complete response rate of 19% for the dabrafenib + trametinib combination. In a pooled analysis that included 563 patients treated with the combination, 34% were alive and 19% were progression-free at 5 years, with median PFS and OS of 11.1 months and 25.9 months, respectively. Of note, patients with normal lactate dehydrogenase (LDH) levels and fewer than 3 sites of metastatic disease were more likely to achieve responses of prolonged duration and to be alive at 5 years.[24,25]

In the coBRIM study, 495 patients with previously untreated BRAF-mutant, advanced melanoma were randomly assigned to vemurafenib (960 mg twice daily continuously, on days 1–28) plus cobimetinib (60 mg daily on days 1–21, followed by a 7-day interval off cobimetinib) in 28-day cycles, or to vemurafenib plus placebo. In an analysis from the 4-year extended follow-up, the gains in OS with combined blockade were confirmed (median OS: 22.5 vs 17.4 months; $P = .005$), with 34.7% alive at 5 years. The incidence of grade 3 to 5 AEs was 77%.[26] The 5-year data of BRAF + MEK inhibitors provide reassurance that there is a "tail-of-the-curve" with targeted therapy as well as immunotherapy. Five-year PFS and OS rates of BRAF + MEK and anti–PD-1 agents appear similar.

The third doublet of BRAF and MEK inhibitors, encorafenib and binimetinib, was investigated in the randomized, phase 3 COLUMBUS trial. A total of 577 patients were randomly assigned to the combination (n = 192), single-agent encorafenib (n = 194), or single-agent vemurafenib (n = 191). The ORR, median PFS, and median OS among patients treated with the combination were 64% (following central review), 14.9 months and 33.6 months. Interestingly, encorafenib and binimetinib resulted in a more favorable toxicity profile, with an incidence of grade 3 to 4 AEs of 64%, versus

67% with single-agent encorafenib, and 66% with single-agent vemurafenib.[27] This is especially notable because the encorafenib dose of 450 mg was higher in combination with binimetinib than as monotherapy (encorafenib 300 mg daily).

Activity of Combinations in Patients with Central Nervous System Metastases

One of the challenges with combination therapy is appropriate patient selection, and there is a general belief that combinations may be most effective in patients with harder-to-treat disease. One such population involves patients with central nervous system (CNS) metastases. Historically, median survival for patients with CNS metastases was approximately 4 months, and influenced by age, functional status, and activity of extracranial disease.[28,29]

Three prospective studies have tested various approved combinations for patients with CNS metastases. The COMBI-MB study was an open-label phase 2 study of dabrafenib and trametinib at standard doses administered to 125 BRAF-mutant patients with CNS involvement, allocated in 4 separate cohorts. In the cohort of asymptomatic patients with BRAFV600E-mutant melanoma (n = 76), 58% achieved an intracranial response. Despite this high intracranial response rate, the investigator-assessed PFS was only 5.6 months, and only 19% of the patients remained progression-free at 12 months. The toxicity profile was consistent with previous studies of dabrafenib and trametinib.[30]

In 2 separate studies, the ABC trial and CheckMate-204 study, the combination of ipilimumab 3 mg/kg and nivolumab 1 mg/kg administered every 3 weeks for 4 doses, followed by single-agent nivolumab, resulted in intracranial activity similar to those observed in patients with exclusively extracranial disease.[31,32] The intracranial ORR was approximately 50% to 60% in selected, asymptomatic patients not requiring systemic steroids, and the rate of PFS at 9 months was almost 60%. No new safety signals were identified in patients with intracranial disease. Of note, single-agent nivolumab resulted in objective responses in only 20% of asymptomatic patients treated in the monotherapy arm in the ABC trial, suggesting the incorporation of ipilimumab substantially adds efficacy on top of anti–PD-1 alone for patients with brain metastases.[31]

Despite the activity of the combination of nivolumab + ipilimumab and dabrafenib and trametinib in selected patients with intracranial disease, these results cannot be generalized to all patients in clinical practice who have CNS metastases. Efficacy in patients who require steroids or are otherwise symptomatic is believed to be low, highlighting the unmet need for more efficacious approaches for these individuals. Follow-up time remains short in these CNS metastasis trials as well, compared with the 5-year follow-up data in prior registrational trials of these agents.

COMBINATIONS OF IMMUNOTHERAPY AND MITOGEN-ACTIVATED PROTEIN KINASE PATHWAY TARGETED THERAPY

Supported by preclinical evidence suggesting a potential interaction between the MAPK pathway and modulation of the tumor immune microenvironment and immune responses through T-cell activation, signaling and trafficking, and increased expression of melanoma antigens in the setting of MAPK pathway inhibition,[33,34] several trials were launched to test combinations of ICB blockade with BRAF ± MEK inhibitors. Unfortunately, combinations of MAPK pathway inhibitors with ipilimumab were found to have toxicity issues, but given their lower rates of toxicity, PD1/PDL1 agents were found to be more favorable combinatorial partners.[35,36]

Encouraging disease control rates approaching 100% in early-phase studies with triplet combinations (BRAF and MEK inhibitors in combination with an anti–PD-1 or PD-L1 agents) in BRAF-mutant melanoma prompted a rapid development of larger, randomized studies investigating whether adding PD-1 or PD-L1 improves the efficacy of BRAF + MEK alone.[37,38] In the phase 2, placebo-controlled, randomized part of the KEYNOTE-022 study, patients with BRAFV600 E/K-mutant melanoma were randomly assigned to dabrafenib and trametinib or a triplet combination with the addition of pembrolizumab; the trial did not meet its primary endpoint and failed to demonstrate a statistically significant improvement in PFS, despite a median PFS of 16.0 m in the triplet arm versus 10.3 m with dabrafenib and trametinib alone.[39] Longer-term follow-up from this study will be important to know whether benefits of triplet therapy increase over time.

The largest randomized trial conducted to date exploring the triplet strategy was recently presented. The IMspire 150 (TRILOGY) was a phase 3, double-blind, placebo-controlled study, in which patients with BRAFV600E-mutation-positive advanced melanoma were randomized to the combination of vemurafenib and cobimetinib at standard doses plus placebo or, following a run-in period of 28 days, to vemurafenib 720 mg twice daily continuously, cobimetinib 60 mg daily for 21 days, and atezolizumab 840 mg administered intravenously every 14 days.[40] The trial met its primary endpoint by demonstrating a significant improvement in investigator-assessed PFS favoring the triplet combination (median PFS: 15.1 m vs 10.6 m; $P = .0249$); OS data were immature at the time of this primary analysis. Interestingly, and somewhat different from the preliminary findings from early-phase clinical trials, ORRs were similar (66.3% with vemurafenib, cobimetinib and atezolizumab vs 65.0% with vemurafenib, cobimetinib and placebo); there was no significant increase in the incidence of serious treatment-related AEs. A similar trial using the triplet combination of the anti–PD-1 agent spartalizumab (PDR-001), dabrafenib and trametinib has completed accrual and results are awaited (NCT02967692). One important consideration with all of these triplet trials is that none include protocol mandated cross-over to a PD1/PDL1 agent at time of progression in the BRAF + MEK alone group as would be pursued in routine clinical practice. Therefore, even though PFS favors triplet therapy, clinicians and health care systems may still prefer sequential use of BRAF + MEK and immunotherapy (or vice versa) as it remains unclear whether OS will be improved with upfront triplet therapy versus sequential administration of these agents.

While BRAF-mutant melanoma has been the focus to study MAPK pathway inhibitors and immunotherapy, the activity of combined MAPK pathway inhibition (MEK inhibition) and ICB blockade was also investigated in patients with BRAF wild-type tumors, with disappointing results. In the phase 3, randomized IMspire 170 trial, there was no significant improvement in PFS, OS, or ORR with the combination of cobimetinib and atezolizumab in comparison with single-agent pembrolizumab (median PFS – primary endpoint: 5.5 m vs 5.7 m; $P = .295$). Why this study was negative is unclear. It could have been due to the low activity of MEK inhibitors in BRAF wild-type melanoma, differences between PD-L1 and PD-1 inhibition in melanoma, or from immunologic effects of MEK inhibition, which may have been detrimental to antitumor immunity. Nonetheless, this result was similar to another randomized study in colorectal cancer in which the combination of MEK and PD-L1 inhibition was not found to be as effective as hoped.[41]

OTHER IMMUNOTHERAPY COMBINATIONS

In addition to anti–CTLA-4 and anti–PD-1 immunotherapies, additional combinatorial agents are being evaluated to enhance antigen processing and presentation, inhibit other T-cell checkpoints, and provide immunologically beneficial cytokines with the goal of increasing an antitumor immune response. T-VEC was approved by the FDA based on the results of a phase 3 trial in which patients with stage IIIB-IV melanoma were treated with intratumoral injections of T-VEC. T-VEC resulted in improved durable responses when compared with GM-CSF alone.[5] The potential for combining T-VEC and systemic ICB has been tested in clinical trials, with promising results and an encouraging safety profile. A randomized study compared the combination of T-VEC and ipilimumab with ipilimumab alone in 198 patients with unresectable stage IIIB to IV melanoma. The use of the combination resulted in a significant improvement in ORR (39% vs 19%; $P = .002$), with responses in lesions that did not receive T-VEC injections.[42] Using a similar approach, T-VEC was combined with pembrolizumab in a phase 1b study including 21 patients; 57.1% achieved an objective response, including 23.8% confirmed complete responses.[43] Although of interest, given challenges interpreting efficacy of combinatorial strategies in small, single-arm studies, we await randomized data and answers to the question of whether T-VEC improves the efficacy of pembrolizumab in the ongoing phase 3, MASTERKEY-265 clinical trial (NCT02263508).

In the field of combined immunotherapy approaches, the activity of combinations of anti–PD-1 agents with agents that target the lymphocyte-activation gene 3 (LAG-3) checkpoint and the interleukin-2 (IL-2) pathway (bempegaldesleukin) are currently in randomized phase 3 studies. LAG-3 is a negative regulator of T-cell function. Relatlimab, an anti–LAG-3 monoclonal antibody, demonstrated activity in a phase I/IIa study in combination with nivolumab in immunotherapy refractory patients and is currently being investigated in a randomized, phase II/III study in treatment-naïve patients in combination with nivolumab versus nivolumab alone (NCT03470922).[44]

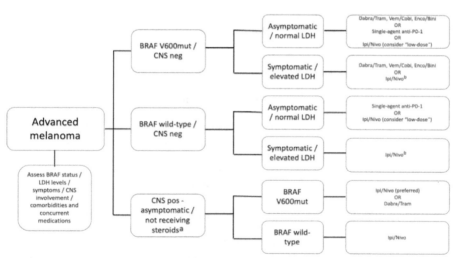

Fig. 1. Overview of proposed treatment algorithms involving combinatorial approaches for patients with advanced melanoma. "low-dose", ipilimumab 1 mg/kg + nivolumab 3 mg/kg; Bini, binimetinib; Cobi, cobimetinib; Dabra, dabrafenib; Enco, encorafenib; Ipi/Nivo, ipilimumab 3 mg/kg + nivolumab 1 mg/kg; Tram, trametinib; Vem, vemurafenib. [a]For patients with symptomatic CNS metastases or using steroids, the optimal approach remains unclear. [b]In these scenarios, single-agent anti–PD-1 is also an acceptable alternative, particularly in select situations (eg, underlying autoimmune diseases, comorbidities).

Bempegaldesleukin is a pegylated IL-2 agonist with preferential binding to the IL-2 receptor's beta-gamma subunit as opposed to the alpha subunit. This preferential binding is hypothesized to lead to more T-effector proliferation with less immunosuppressive T-regulatory cell expansion. In early-phase nonrandomized studies, bempegaldesleukin in combination with nivolumab resulted in encouraging antitumor activity, but similar to relatlimab, randomized data are needed.[45] A phase 3 study testing bempegaldesleukin + nivolumab versus nivolumab alone is accruing patients (NCT-3635983).

DISCUSSION AND SUMMARY

Robust advances confirmed across several clinical trials have led to the approval of multiple therapies for the treatment of patients with advanced melanoma, improving life expectancy in profound ways. Examples of these agents incorporated into clinical practice in recent years include ICB blockade with anti–CTLA-4 and anti–PD-1 monoclonal antibodies, targeted therapies represented by BRAF and MEK inhibitors and the oncolytic viral therapy, T-VEC.

Despite the improvements produced by single-agent regimens, combinatorial approaches are currently considered among the standard treatment options and have substantially improved the outcomes for patients with advanced melanoma. For those with tumors harboring a BRAF mutation and candidates for targeted therapy, the combined use of BRAF and MEK inhibitors has consistently replaced single-agent vemurafenib or dabrafenib. In the field of immunotherapy, single-agent anti–PD-1 with nivolumab or pembrolizumab alone or the nivolumab + ipilimumab combination is a reasonable treatment approach.

This multiplication in the number of treatment alternatives favorably translates into a welcome growing complexity of treatment algorithms for patients who present with advanced melanoma (**Fig. 1**). Unfortunately, the only established biomarker continues to be the BRAF-mutation status, as the expression of PD-L1 has not been shown to be a useful biomarker in melanoma to select treatment. The best treatment to be given upfront for BRAF-mutant patients remains to be determined, and results of ongoing studies looking at the best sequence and combinations of BRAF/MEK inhibition and ICB are eagerly awaited. More recently, with the possibility of using triplet combinations composed of BRAF and MEK inhibitors in combination with PD1/PDL1 ICB blockers, a relevant clinical question that is beginning to emerge is which patients with BRAF-mutant tumors will be the best candidates for immunotherapy alone versus the combination of immunotherapy with targeted therapies versus targeted therapy alone. OS data from randomized phase 3 studies with high rates of PD1 ICB use after progression in the BRAF + MEK alone control group are needed to fully understand where triplet therapy will reside in the treatment algorithm.

Variables that directly influence the choice for first-line therapies encompass, in addition to the BRAF-mutation status, the presence or absence of brain metastases, serum LDH levels, the burden of disease, presence of symptoms, and additional factors that include barriers to accessing care, social support, comorbidities (eg, underlying autoimmune diseases, history of solid-organ transplantation) and the use of concurrent medications.[46] For patients with normal LDH levels, limited disease burden, and no CNS involvement, long-term benefit can be achieved with both BRAF/MEK inhibitors and ICB blockade, as demonstrated by recent updates of KEYNOTE-006, CheckMate-067, COMBI-v, and COMBI-d studies. For this subgroup, the favorable safety profile demonstrated by single-agent anti–PD-1 in comparison with ipilimumab + nivolumab must be considered, although the latter regimen can be considered due to the potential benefits in response rate and PFS, particularly adopting ipilimumab at "low doses" (1 mg/kg). In parallel, this is also the subgroup that does best with combined BRAF/MEK inhibitors. In this setting of favorable prognostic factors, comorbidities, the spectrum of AEs, preference for oral or intravenous therapy, and the potential of drug interactions may contribute to the choice of treatment, as targeted agents may share metabolic pathways with concomitant medications through the cytochrome P450 complex. Based on the results of contemporary, noncomparative trials with a limited number of patients, nivolumab + ipilimumab remains the treatment of choice for those presenting with asymptomatic CNS involvement, and can be considered for individuals with BRAF wild-type melanoma with elevated LDH, multiple sites of disease (particularly in the presence of bone or liver involvement) or symptomatic patients who may have an opportunity for only 1 line of systemic therapy.

In summary, combinatorial approaches represent a new standard in the management of patients with advanced melanoma, and an expansion in the plethora of potential combinations is expected in the coming years. Nevertheless, translational research, effective biomarkers, and future clinical trials are warranted to address the large body of questions that remain to be answered, and to enable rational, patient-centered, and cost-effective incorporation of novel approaches.

CLINICS CARE POINTS

- Combinatorial approaches in melanoma hold the potential to enhance antitumor activity and, in specific scenarios, mitigate toxicities
- Single-agent nivolumab or pembrolizumab result in response rates of approximately 40%, with the possibility of long-term benefits; single-agent T-VEC has a limited role in the first-line setting; single-agent BRAF inhibitors are no longer a standard treatment due to superiority of BRAF + mitogen-activated protein kinase kinase MEK inhibitor combinations
- Combinatorial approaches currently approved for clinical use include ipilimumab and nivolumab and, for patients with melanoma harboring a BRAF mutation, doublets of BRAF and MEK inhibitors vemurafenib and cobimetinib, dabrafenib and trametinib and encorafenib and binimetinib
- Across several randomized, clinical trials, combinations of BRAF/MEK inhibitors resulted in superior outcomes in comparison to single-agent BRAF inhibitors, without an increase in the absolute incidence of adverse events
- The combination of ipilimumab and nivolumab results in an increased objective response rate at the risk of an increased frequency of immune-related adverse events and treatment discontinuations. No statistically significant improvement in overall survival over single-agent anti–PD-1 alone has been demonstrated to date with this combination; treatment decisions for patients with advanced melanoma are driven by BRAF-mutation status, presence or absence of central nervous system metastases, disease burden, symptoms, serum lactate dehydrogenase levels, comorbidities, and concurrent medications, among other factors.

ACKNOWLEDGMENTS

There was no specific funding received for this article.

DISCLOSURE

R.R. Munhoz: research involvement: BMS, Lilly, Merck, MSD, Novartis, Roche; honoraria: Bayer, BMS, Merck, MSD, Novartis, Roche, Sanofi; travel grants: BMS, Novartis, Sanofi. M.A. Postow: consulting fees from 2015-present: BMS, Merck, Array Bio-Pharma, Novartis, Incyte, NewLink Genetics, Aduro; honoraria: BMS and Merck; institutional Support: RGenix, Infinity, BMS, Merck, Array BioPharma, Novartis, AstraZeneca.

REFERENCES

1. Siegel RL, Miller KD, Jemal A. Cancer Statistics, 2020. CA Cancer J Clin 2020; 70:7–30.
2. Glazer AM, Winkelmann RR, Farberg AS, et al. Analysis of trends in US melanoma incidence and mortality. JAMA Dermatol 2017;153(2):225–6.
3. Chen DS, Mellman I. Elements of cancer immunity and the cancer-immune set-point. Nature 2017;541(7637):321–30.
4. Luke JJ, Flaherty KT, Ribas A, et al. Targeted agents and immunotherapies: optimizing outcomes in melanoma. Nat Rev Clin Oncol 2017;14(8):463–82.
5. Andtbacka RHI, Collichio F, Harrington KJ, et al. Final analyses of OPTiM: a randomized phase III trial of talimogene laherparepvec versus granulocyte-macrophage colony-stimulating factor in unresectable stage III–IV melanoma. J Immunother Cancer 2019;7(1):145.
6. Topalian SL, Hodi FS, Brahmer JR, et al. Five-year survival and correlates among patients with advanced melanoma, renal cell carcinoma, or non-small cell lung cancer treated with nivolumab. JAMA Oncol 2019;10:1411–20.
7. Hamid O, Robert C, Daud A, et al. Five-year survival outcomes for patients with advanced melanoma treated with pembrolizumab in KEYNOTE-001. Ann Oncol 2019;30(4):582–8.
8. Ascierto PA, Long GV, Robert C, et al. Survival outcomes in patients with previously-untreated BRAF wild-type advanced melanoma treated with nivolumab therapy. Three-year follow-up of a randomized phase 3 trial. JAMA Oncol 2019;5(2):187–94.
9. Larkin J, Chiarion-Sileni V, Gonzalez R, et al. Five-year survival with combined nivolumab + ipilimumab in advanced melanoma. N Engl J Med 2019;381:1535–46.
10. Robert C, Ribas A, Schachter J, et al. Pembrolizumab versus ipilimumab in advanced melanoma (KEYNOTE-006): post-hoc 5-year results from an open-label, multicentre, randomized, controlled, phase 3 study. Lancet Oncol 2019; 20(9):1239–51.
11. McCarthur GA, Chapman PB, Robert C, et al. Safety and efficacy of vemurafenib in *BRAFV600E* and *BRAFV600K* mutation-positive melanoma (BRIM-3): extended follow-up of a phase 3, randomised, open-label study. Lancet Oncol 2014;15: 323–32.
12. Hauschild A, Ascierto PA, Schadendorf D, et al. Long-term outcomes in patients with BRAF V600-mutant metastatic melanoma receiving dabrafenib monotherapy: Analysis from phase 2 and 3 clinical trials. Eur J Cancer 2020;125:114–20.
13. Wolchok JD, Kluger H, Callahan MK, et al. Nivolumab plus ipilimumab in advanced melanoma. N Engl J Med 2013;369:122–33.
14. Curran MA, Montalvo W, Yagita H, et al. PD-1 and CTLA-4 combination blockade expands infiltrating T cells and reduces regulatory T and myeloid cells within B16 melanoma tumors. Proc Natl Acad Sci U S A 2010;107(9):4275–80.

15. Wolchok JD, Neyns B, Linette G, et al. Ipilimumab monotherapy in patients with pretreated advanced melanoma: a randomised, double-blind, multicentre, phase 2, dose-ranging study. Lancet Oncol 2010;11(2):155–64.

16. Ascierto PA, Del Vecchio M, Robert C, et al. Ipilimumab 10 mg/kg versus ipilimumab 3 mg/kg in patients with unresectable or metastatic melanoma: a randomised, double-blind, multicentre, phase 3 trial. Lancet Oncol 2017;18(5):611–22.

17. Hodi FS, O'Day SJ, McDermott DF, et al. Improved survival with ipilimumab in patients with metastatic melanoma. N Engl J Med 2010;363:711–23.

18. Postow MA, Chesney J, Pavlick AC, et al. Nivolumab + ipilimumab versus ipilimumab in untreated melanoma. N Engl J Med 2015;372:2006–17.

19. Hodi FS, Chesney J, Pavlick AC, et al. Combined nivolumab + ipilimumab versus ipilimumab alone in patients with advanced melanoma: 2-year overall survival outcomes in a multicentre, randomised, controlled, phase 2 trial. Lancet Oncol 2016;17(11):1558–68.

20. Larkin J, Chiarion-Sileni V, Gonzalez R, et al. Combined nivolumab + ipilimumab or monotherapy in untreated melanoma. N Engl J Med 2015;373:23–34.

21. Long GV, Atkinson V, Cebon JS, et al. Standard-dose pembrolizumab in combination with reduced-dose ipilimumab for patients with advanced melanoma (KEYNOTE-029): an open-label, phase 1b trial. Lancet Oncol 2017;18(9):1202–10.

22. Lebbé C, Meyer N, Mortier L, et al. Evaluation of two dosing regimens for nivolumab in combination with ipilimumab in patients with advanced melanoma: results from the phase IIIb/Iv CheckMate 511 trial. J Clin Oncol 2019;37(11):867–75.

23. Rizos H, Menzies AM, Pupo GM, et al. BRAF inhibitor resistance mechanisms in metastatic melanoma: spectrum and clinical impact. Clin Cancer Res 2014;20(7):1965–77.

24. Long GV, Grob JJ, Nathan P, et al. Factors predictive of response, disease progression, and overall survival after dabrafenib and trametinib combination treatment: a pooled analysis of individual patient data from randomised trials. Lancet Oncol 2016;17(12):1743–54.

25. Robert C, Grob JJ, Stroyakovskiy D, et al. Five-year outcomes with dabrafenib plus trametinib in metastatic melanoma. N Engl J Med 2019;381:626–36.

26. Dréno B, Ascierto PA, McCarthur GA, et al. Efficacy and safety of cobimetinibe combined with vemurafenib in patients with BRAFV600 mutation-positive metastatic melanoma: analysis from the 4-year extended follow up of the phase 3 coBRIM study. J Clin Oncol 2018;36(15_suppl):9522.

27. Dummer R, Ascierto PA, Gogas HJ, et al. Overall survival in COLUMBUS: A phase 3 trial of encorafenib (ENCO) plus binimetinib (BINI) vs vemurafenib (VEM) or ENCO in BRAF-mutant-melanoma. J Clin Oncol 2018;36(no 15_suppl):9504.

28. Cagney DN, Martin AM, Catalano PJ, et al. Incidence and prognosis of patients with brain metastases at diagnosis of systemic malignancy: a population-based study. Neuro Oncol 2017;19:1511–21.

29. Sperduto PW, Jiang W, Brown PD, et al. Estimating survival in melanoma patients with brain metastases: an update of the graded prognostic assessment for melanoma using molecular markers (Melanoma-molGPA). Int J Radiat Oncol Biol Phys 2017;99(4):812–6.

30. Davies MA, Saiag P, Robert C, et al. Dabrafenib plus trametinibe in patients with BRAFV600-mutant melanoma brain metastases (COMBI-MB): a multicentre, multicohort, open-label, phase 2 trial. Lancet Oncol 2017;18(7):863–73.

31. Long GV, Atkinson V, Lo S, et al. Combination nivolumab + ipilimumab or nivolumab alone in melanoma brain metastases: a multicentre randomised phase 2 study. Lancet Oncol 2018;19(5):672–81.
32. Tawbi HA, Forsyth PA, Algazi A, et al. Combined nivolumab + ipilimumab in melanoma metastatic to the brain. N Engl J Med 2018;379(8):722–30.
33. Frederick DT, Piris A, Cogdill AP, et al. BRAF inhibition is associated with enhanced melanoma antigen expression and a more favorable tumor microenvironment in patients with metastatic melanoma. Clin Cancer Res 2013;19(5): 1225–31.
34. Hu-Lieskovan S, Mok S, Moreno BH, et al. Improved antitumor activity of immunotherapy with BRAF and MEK inhibitors in BRAFV600E melanoma. Sci Transl Med 2015;7(279):279ra41.
35. Ribas A, Hodi FS, Callahan MK, et al. Hepatotoxicity with combination of vemurafenib and ipilimumab. N Engl J Med 2013;368(4):1365–6.
36. Minor DR, Puzanov I, Callahan MK, et al. Severe gastrointestinal toxicity with administration of trametinib in combination with dabrafenib and ipilimumab. Pigment Cell Melanoma Res 2015;28(5):611–2.
37. Sullivan RJ, Hamid O, Gonzalez R, et al. Atezolizumab plus cobimetinib and vemurafenib in *BRAF*-mutated melanoma patients. Nat Med 2019;25(6):929–35.
38. Ribas A, Lawrence D, Atkinson V, et al. Combined BRAF and MEK inhibition with PD-1 blockade immunotherapy in BRAF-mutant melanoma. Nat Med 2019;25(6): 936–40.
39. Ascierto PA, Ferrucci PF, Fisher R, et al. Dabrafenib, trametinib and pembrolizumab or placebo in BRAF-mutant melanoma. Nat Med 2019;25(6):941–6.
40. Gutzmer R, Stroyakovskiy D, Gogas H, et al. Atezolizumab, vemurafenib, and cobimetinib as first-line treatment for unresectable advanced BRAF V600 mutation-positive melanoma (IMspire150): primary analysis of the randomised, double-blind, placebo-controlled, phase 3 trial. Lancet 2020; 395(10240):1835-44.
41. Eng C, Kim TW, Bendell J, et al. Atezolizumab with or without cobimetinib versus regorafenib in previously treated metastatic colorectal cancer (IMblaze370): a multicentre, open-label, phase 3, randomised, controlled trial. Lancet Oncol 2019;20(6):849–61.
42. Chesney J, Puzanov I, Collichio F, et al. Randomized, Open-label phase II study evaluating the efficacy and safety of talimogenelaherparepvec in combination with ipilimumab versus ipilimumab alone in patients with advanced, unresectable melanoma. J Clin Oncol 2018;36(17):1658–67.
43. Long GV, Dummer R, Ribas A, et al. Efficacy analysis of MASTERKEY-265 phase 1b study of talimogene laherparepvec (T-VEC) and pembrolizumab (pembro) for unresectable stage IIIB-IV melanoma. J Clin Oncol 2016;(34_suppl):9568.
44. Ascierto PA, Melero I, Bhatia S, et al. Initial efficacy of anti-lymphocyte activation gene-3 (anti–LAG-3; BMS-986016) in combination with nivolumab (nivo) in pts with melanoma (MEL) previously treated with anti–PD-1/PD-L1 therapy. J Clin Oncol 2017;35(no 15_suppl):9520.
45. Diab A, Cho D, Papadimitrakopoulou V, et al. NKTR-214 (CD122-biased agonist) plus nivolumab in patients with advanced solid tumors: Preliminary phase 1/2 results of PIVOT. J Clin Oncol 2018;36(no_15_suppl):3006.
46. Seth R, Messersmith H, Kaur V, et al. Systemic therapy for melanoma: ASCO guideline. J Clin Oncol 2020. https://doi.org/10.1200/JCO.20.00198.